. . . .

Your Premature Baby

Everything You Need to Know About the Childbirth, Treatment, and Parenting of Premature Infants

Frank P. Manginello, M.D., and Theresa Foy DiGeronimo

Drawings by Robert E. Myers

John Wiley & Sons, Inc.
New York • Chichester • Brisbane • Toronto • Singapore

Every effort has been made to make this book a thoroughly up-to-date resource, however, you should realize that the field of neonatology is continuously growing and changing. Between the time of writing this book and its publication, a medical advance has been made in the treatment of respiratory distress syndrome (RDS), a lung disease that is the most common cause of death in preemies under 3 pounds. (See Chapter Two.) The U.S. Food and Drug Administration recently approved the use of an artificial surfactant for the treatment of RDS. This substance, which is produced naturally in full-term infants, is often lacking in preemies under 3 pounds, so unless it is supplied artificially, preemies may develop significant respiratory problems. The drug can be used as a prophylactic measure before the baby takes his first breath, or as treatment for a pre-existing lung problem. Although its complete success as a treatment has yet to be determined, its very recent approval for use illustrates the need to use this book as a source of information secondary to your doctor's first-hand, personal advice.

The authors have worked closely together to write this book; the first-person "I" who speaks to you throughout the book is the voice of Dr. Manginello.

ISBN 0 471-53587-7

Printed in the United States of America.

91 92 10 9 8 7 6 5 4 3 2 1

Acknowledgments

. . . .

We would like to acknowledge the medical professionals who willingly gave their time and expertise to help make this book as accurate and up-to-date as possible:

Daniel Adler, M.D.
Child Neurologist
Valley Hospital, Ridgewood, N.J.

Virginia Albertsen-D'Alessandro, R.N., C., M.S.N.
Assistant Director of Nursing Maternal/Child Health
Valley Hospital, Ridgewood, N.J.

Lorraine Burstein, R.N., R.R.T.
Clinical Director of Pediatric Home Care Associates
Garfield, N.J.

Frank DeMaria, Jr., M.D.
Chief of Pediatrics
Valley Hospital, Ridgewood, N.J.

Benjamin Dispenziere, M.D.
Perinatologist
Associate Clinical Professor
University of Medicine and Dentistry of NJ
Newark, N.J.

Joanne Foose, M.T., A.S.C.P.
Medical Technologist
Valley Hospital, Ridgewood, N.J.

Maura Gallagher, M.S.
Perinatal Social Worker/ICN
St. Joseph's Hospital and Medical Center, Paterson, N.J.

Jeffrey R. Greenwald, M.D.
Fellow in Neonatology
St. Peter's Medical Center New Brunswick, N.J.

David V. Habif, Jr., M.D.
Pediatric Radiologist
Teaneck Radiology Center
Teaneck, N.J.

Nina Halstead, R.N., B.S.N.
Head Nursery Nurse
Valley Hospital, Ridgewood, N.J.

Michele Hepp, M.S.W., C.S.W.
Coordinator of Social Work Services
Valley Hospital, Ridgewood, N.J.

Joseph Holahan, M.D.
Chief of Developmental Pediatrics
St. Joseph's Hospital and Medical Center, Paterson, N.J.

Arthur A. Klein, M.D.
Pediatric Cardiologist/Vice-Chairman of Pediatrics
New York Hospital-Cornell University Medical Center

Ronald Lunn, M.A., C.C.C.-Aud.
Audiologist
St. Joseph's Hospital and Medical Center, Paterson, N.J.

Donna E. Nickles, D.O.
Obstetrics and Gynecology
Valley Hospital, Ridgewood, N.J.

Poorvi Patel, M.D.
Chief of Pediatric Neurology
St. Joseph's Hospital and Medical Center, Paterson, N.J.

Leslie Richardson
Medical Secretary
Valley Hospital, Ridgewood, N.J.

Tine K. Williams R.N., C., M.S.N.,
 P.N.P.
Nurse Coordinator ICN Follow-
 up Program
St. Joseph's Hospital and Medical
 Center, Paterson, N.J.

Stuart E. Wunsh, M.D., F.A.C.S.
Pediatric Ophthalmologist
Clifton, N.J.

Of course this book could not have been written if it weren't for the many people who opened their hearts and shared with us the feelings, attitudes, and experiences of families with preemies. Although it is impossible to publically acknowledge each individual person (especially because some have opted in the name of privacy to use pseudonyms) we would now like to thank everyone who gave us their time and shared their stories. We offer a special note of thanks to:

Norma and John Clark and
 Tommy
Lisa and Jack Crilly and Alycia and
 Virginia
Bonnie and George Dzendzel and
 David
Elizabeth and Richard Gordon and
 "Flash"

Bergman and Walter Li and
 Kathleen
Nancy and Bruce Liljegren and
 Dana
Rosalind McGrady and Kevin
Mary Ellen and Tony Zizzi and
 Christine

Contents

· ·

Introduction

Last night, twelve weeks before her due date, Beth gave birth to a baby girl. This morning, she will find herself hurtled into a crash course on prematurity as she and her husband begin their search for information. Their three years' experience parenting their first child will not help them now to answer questions such as: "How is she different from a full-term baby?" "What are all those tubes and wires going into her?" "Why does she need so many doctors?" "How can I bond with a baby I have to leave behind in the hospital?" "What's her prognosis?" "When can she come home?"

Their family and friends will also be at a loss. They may not know what to say or what to do. Should they offer sympathy and a shoulder to cry on? Or, should they offer congratulations and remain optimistic? The grandparents may remember what a premature birth used to mean. They'll recall horrible stories of frail preemies who eventually died or lived with awful physical defects and handicaps. What should they say? Their only source of information may be the 1945 book *Baby And Child Care* by Dr. Benjamin Spock that's still on their bookshelf. It explains how to keep a premature baby in a cardboard box lined with newspapers and heated with bricks, bags of sand, or even small boulders that have been preheated in the oven, and how to make a wooden peaked incubator and heat it with a 25- or 40-watt light bulb. They'll quickly realize that they have little practical advice to offer.

How will Beth and her husband find the information they need? If they look in bookstores and libraries, they may get outdated (but still in-print) books that present inaccurate and frightening statistics about premature birth. They may be misled and offered little hope for their baby's normal development under circumstances that today do not at all indicate imminent retardation or physical disabilities.

What Beth and her husband need to know is that the survival rate for premature babies born after 28 weeks in utero, and the prognosis for their healthy, normal development, has improved dramatically in just the last few years. New procedures, equipment, medications, and a wealth of research and knowledge have all combined to give these babies survival rates bordering on 90 percent. The medical professionals involved in their baby's care will explain all these new advantages and they'll give them all the facts. But when Beth and her husband mix these facts with the rumors, old wives' tales, and outdated information, and then stir in their own worries, concerns, and stressed emotional state, the facts may not rise to the top, and they probably won't have the mental energy to sort them out. For many parents of premature babies, the search for information leads only to a muddled mess.

A few months ago I was explaining a medical procedure to a young mother when she cut me off to confess, "I think I understand what you're telling me, but when my husband arrives and I try to explain it to him, I know I won't remember all the details; I know I won't be able to answer his questions. Can you write all this down for me?" Now, for the parents of the three hundred thousand or so premature babies born each year in this country, I've written it all down in this book. It contains accurate, up-to-date information that you can absorb slowly, carefully, and thoughtfully. This book is not meant to take the place of close communication between you and your baby's health care providers; it is written to enhance your understanding of what they tell you. The professionals involved in your baby's care will give you in-depth explanations of his health and of all necessary procedures and treatments. But from my years of working with the parents of preemies, I know that in your heightened emotional state, the desire to listen and understand may not always keep up with your ability to pay attention. This book will give you the kind of reinforcement that will help those facts "sink in."

In the weeks and months after a premature birth, there will probably be little time to sit back, put your feet up, and read a good book. Knowing that, I have organized this book in a way that will help you quickly find specific pieces of information—those appropriate to your particular situation. Each chapter can be read out of sequence as it meets your needs. If a term or procedure was explained more fully in another section, you will be given that page reference, and the Glossary in the back of the book will also be a useful resource for finding definitions of medical terms.

If you are reading this book in advance of your baby's birth, the information in Chapter One on premature labor and delivery may be of particular interest to you right now. If you have already delivered prematurely, you should note in the Contents that the three levels of prematurity are presented in three separate chapters. Find the one that describes your baby's age and weight and ignore the others. (If your baby's weight is in one category and his age is in another, the category describing his weight will be most appropriate.) By doing this, you won't get misleading or inappropriate information. Very often parents come to me with misinformation that scares or confuses them. They have questions about things like surgical procedures, prematurity-related blindness, and radiation exposure. Once we sit down and sort it out, they often realize that it has nothing to do with their baby's particular level of prematurity.

Chapter Three presents a description of medical complications that are sometimes caused by a premature birth.

This chapter has the potential to scare parents with all the frightening things that *might* go wrong. Don't let it do this to you. Use this chapter only as a reference source to back up and explain what your baby's doctors tell you. Don't take each problem and impose it on your baby. A complication's potential impact on your baby's well-being can be understood only in the context of your child's birth age and weight, the information your baby's doctor shares with you, and your preemie's status as a human being unique from all others. Just as some full-term babies are born with medical complications that cannot be generalized for all newborns, so it is with preemies and their health problems.

Even as you sort out the facts and begin to understand your baby's special needs, you may find yourself floundering in a whirl of mixed emotions. If that happens to you, read Chapter Seven. It will help you see that your feelings are normal and are to be expected. It will show you that other parents have felt the same way as you, and it will explain the progression of feelings that commonly accompany a premature birth.

Then, when you are ready to roll up your sleeves and become actively involved in the day-to-day care of your baby, use Chapter Eight as your guide. It will encourage you to step forward to take your rightful place as a member of the primary-care team responsible for your baby's growth and development. It will give you practical tips that will make the job of parenting through an incubator just a bit easier. It will help you master the transition from hospital to home baby care.

In this age of modern medical science, it's sometimes difficult to understand why your questions about your baby's future can't be answered immediately after his birth. But the fact is, there are some aspects of human development we don't know everything about yet, and there are some questions that can be answered only in time. This is true even of the questions that parents of full-term babies ask. Pediatricians may offer educated guesses in answer to questions such as: "When will she grow some hair?" "When will he sleep through the night?" "When will she get her first tooth?" But they can't guarantee the answers will be right. Other questions have no immediate answers at all. Questions such as, "Will this baby have colic like my first baby?" "Will he be tall like his grandfather?" "Do you think she'll develop food allergies?" all belong to the wait-and-see category of child rearing.

It may be very hard to wait and see what will happen to your preemie. But you'll make this difficult time even more difficult by looking for answers to questions about the distant future. Ask the doctors how your baby is doing *today.* Find out all you can about the procedures and treatments he needs *now.* Learn how you can help him and care for him in whatever circumstances he experiences at present. Don't jump ahead and read about all the complications known to modern medicine; don't seek out material on the death of infants, and don't listen to people who tell you sad or painful stories. Make yourself concentrate on being the best parent you can be *today.* Then tomorrow, start again.

You'll notice that discussions of death and severe birth defects are not included in this book. This is not meant to deny the fact that some infants die and others are left with extreme physical and/or mental handicaps. But the parents of these babies (both premature and full-term) need different kinds of information and support than can be adequately offered within the scope of this book. Also, this kind of information would serve no constructive purpose for parents of the vast majority of preemies who will survive in good health. Human nature being what it is, these parents may first look for the worst that could possibly happen. Including a chapter on death and handicaps would not give them facts pertinent to their baby, nor the support and encouragement they need and deserve. This book is about life and growth. It is about the miracles that modern medicine now make routine. It's about beautiful children who are born too soon, and it's about the parents who love them, care for them, and raise them, one day at a time.

Chapter One

The Birth of a Preemie

W hen a woman goes into premature labor, her first
question is, of course, "Why is this happening?"
Sometimes there is an exact identifiable reason,
but other times no one can say for sure. This book opens
with a discussion of some of the possible reasons behind
the early birth of your child because the labor, delivery,
and birth are all part of the parenting-a-preemie package.
The information is presented briefly and it is not meant to
take the place of proper medical care, but it will give you
a base of general information from which to learn more
about your baby and his needs, and your role in his care.

Some specific, recognizable conditions and problems that
have been associated with premature delivery include:

1. a previous miscarriage or premature birth
Exactly why obstetric history affects future pregnancies
is not fully understood, but statistically it is known that a
woman who has had one premature delivery has a 20 to
30 percent chance of having another. If a woman has had

two premature births, some researchers report that her chance of having a third preemie jumps as high as 70 percent.

2. two or more abortions

Studies have shown that multiple abortions increase the risk of premature delivery. The reasons for this are unclear.

3. a history of kidney disease

Women who have kidney disease during pregnancy may develop significant complications that can endanger the fetus. A urinary tract infection, for example, may cause a high fever, which, if left untreated, can cause premature labor. Also, kidney damage may cause an increase in blood pressure, which can damage the placenta (a vascular organ that lines the uterine wall, attaches to the umbilical cord, and delivers nourishment to the fetus), cause fetal distress, decrease the fetal oxygen supply, and/or cause poor growth patterns. These conditions have been known to bring on premature labor or necessitate premature delivery.

4. abnormal anatomy of the uterus

There are three abnormalities that most commonly influence the chances of a premature delivery:

(a) a weakened cervix (the lower part of the uterus that opens into the birth canal), which may open before the thirty-eighth week of gestation without uterine contractions

(b) a uterus that is indented on top, causing it to be heart-shaped rather than the normal pear shape

(c) a uterus that has separated into two parts, or is partially divided by a wall of tissue.

5. pregnancy before age sixteen or after age thirty-four

There are many possible reasons why age may cause premature labor—any one of them might be true, but none has been absolutely proven. It's plausible that young girls have a high incidence of prematurity because many of them do not get proper, ongoing prenatal care. It's also possible that their growing bodies compete with the fetus for necessary nutrients, or perhaps they consume more alcohol, cigarettes, and drugs than older women.

It is thought that some older women deliver prematurely because they are more prone to the diseases that can negatively affect a pregnancy, such as hypertension, diabetes, and heart and kidney disease. It's also possible that older women have an increased intake of alcohol and cigarette smoke, exercise less frequently, and are more likely to be under- or overweight than younger women. All of these things can influence their ability to carry to term.

6. exposure to DES (diethylstilbestrol)

If a pregnant woman took the synthetic estrogen hormone DES during her pregnancy to avoid having a miscarriage (as was commonly prescribed in the 1950s and 1960s), a daughter born of that pregnancy may now be at risk for having a premature delivery because she may have structural problems in her uterus, cervix, or vagina, or be predisposed to vaginal cancer.

In addition to these six known conditions that place a woman at high risk for a premature birth, there are also a number of factors and medical complications that can come into play during the pregnancy and put a woman at risk for premature delivery. The most common of these factors are:

1. placental abruption

This is a condition in which the placenta prematurely pulls away from the wall of the uterus, causing painful vaginal bleeding and premature delivery. It is often associated with high blood pressure and cigarette smoking.

2. placenta previa

This is a condition in which the placenta covers the cervical opening of the birth canal. This can cause painless vaginal bleeding, and because it can be life-threatening to both the mother and the fetus, it may necessitate an emergency cesarean delivery.

3. abnormal amounts of amniotic fluid

Too much amniotic fluid in the uterine cavity (a condition called polyhydramnios) puts extra pressure on the uterus and may cause premature birth. This happens more frequently in multiple pregnancies and in pregnancies complicated by diabetes, or when there is an abnormality in the fetus, such as an intestinal obstruction. Too little amniotic fluid (a condition called oligohydramnios) can inhibit normal fetal growth. It can be caused by placental abnormalities, toxemia or preeclampsia, or fetal renal obstruction problems. Both too much and too little amniotic fluid are associated with premature birth as well as a variety of birth defects.

4. uterine fibroids

Uterine fibroids are benign (noncancerous) muscular growths in the wall of the uterus. They are commonly found in women in their thirties and forties. These growths can cause placental abruption, intrauterine growth retardation, and premature birth.

5. toxemia/preeclampsia

Toxemia and preeclampsia are used interchangeably to describe a condition characterized by high blood pressure, fluid retention, and protein in the urine. Other symptoms may include rapid weight gain, headaches, and eye problems. This condition can cause a reduction in the amount of blood flow through the placenta, which slows down the delivery of vital nutrients. If left untreated, it will progress to eclampsia, which is life-threatening to both the mother and child. Toxemia is more likely to develop in women who have preexisting hypertension, diabetes, and/or kidney disease.

6. ruptured membranes

If the bag of amniotic fluid surrounding the baby ruptures at or after 34 weeks gestation, a woman will deliver her baby shortly after the rupture. If, however, the membrane ruptures before 34 weeks gestation, the attending physician will try to hold off her delivery for as long as possible. But, because the fetus is exposed to life-threatening infections without the bag of water and mucus plug as protection, if the mother develops a fever (or any other sign of infection) delivery is imperative.

7. abdominal surgery

Surgery that directly stimulates the uterus may cause premature contractions and subsequent birth. Therefore, a woman who needs an elective surgical procedure may find that her doctors will try to reschedule or postpone the surgery in the hope of safeguarding the fetus and keeping him in utero as long as possible. However, the effect on the pregnancy of emergency surgery on organs other than the uterus depends on the proximity of the organ to the uterus and the gestational age of the baby.

8. multiple births

Twins, triplets, and so on are ten times more likely to be born prematurely than are single births. The physical stress placed on the uterus makes it prone to many complications such as placenta previa and abruption, polyhydramnios, and premature rupture of the membranes.

9. heavy smoking

The toxins in cigarette smoke pass through the placenta to the fetus. Perhaps this is why women who smoke more than ten cigarettes a day have a higher incidence of placental abruption and previa. It seems that the more a woman smokes, the more likely it is to cause premature labor.

10. insufficient prenatal care

Many of the above complications can be diagnosed and treated early in a pregnancy to eliminate or lessen the chances of premature birth. A woman who does not have the benefit of early medical intervention, as well as necessary information, guidance, and nutritional counseling, is more likely to deliver prematurely than one who receives appropriate obstetric care.

Women who have any of these high-risk conditions can often prepare in advance for the possibility of a premature birth. Knowing what to expect, knowing who can offer you and your baby the best care, and knowing where you can get that care are the best ways to ease the difficulties of premature birth. In addition to reading this book, talk to your obstetrician and look into the possibility of consulting with a perinatologist (a medical doctor who specializes in the complications of high-risk pregnancy, labor, and delivery). This doesn't necessarily mean you will have to change doctors; very often your obstetrician will continue your routine care, while the perinatologist will periodically check for problems, do necessary and appropriate testing, and perhaps arrange for a home monitor that can alert you to the onset of early labor. You should also find out the hospital affiliation of the obstetrician and perinatologist and arrange to give birth there so that you and your baby will receive immediate and intensive care if necessary, and so you won't have to be separated from your baby, who may need the kind of care available only in the intensive care nurseries of selected hospitals.

Knowing in advance that you are at risk for premature labor improves the chances that, with medical help, you'll be able to carry your baby closer to term. But the high-risk factors listed above account for only approximately 40 percent of premature deliveries. When the other 60 percent of the women who deliver prematurely ask, "Why is this happening?" the only honest answer their obstetricians can give is "I don't know." For these women with no medical complications, no poor health habits, no history of obstetric or medical problems, the premature birth of their baby comes as a complete surprise. Most women who deliver prematurely without warning experience a labor and delivery similar to Sue's:

"I was having a wonderful pregnancy. I hadn't had any morning sickness, or feelings of extreme fatigue, or backaches, or any of the other discomforts I was expecting. In fact, I felt great! I had been to my obstetrician on Tuesday afternoon for my six-month checkup. She said everything was fine. The baby was the right size; his heartbeat was strong; my weight gain was just right, and my blood pressure was normal.

"The following Saturday I noticed some spots of blood on my underwear so I called my doctor. She wasn't in the office, but her nurse said it was probably nothing to worry about. She suggested that maybe I had overexerted myself and it might help if I stayed off my feet for a while. That sounded plausible to me, and so without much concern, I sat back with my feet up for the rest of the day. That night the spotting turned into heavy bleeding. Even though I wasn't in any pain or feeling any contractions, I knew something was very wrong. I called my doctor and told her about the increased bleeding, and reminded her how quickly my last labor and delivery had progressed. We agreed to meet at the hospital.

"In the labor and delivery area, I was strapped to a monitor that recorded the baby's heartbeat and the start of mild contractions. By the time my obstetrician decided to admit me into the hospital, I was so worried about my baby that my heart was pounding, my body was shaking, and I could barely get my questions out past the lump in my throat. I couldn't believe this was happening to me. I wasn't supposed to be in this birthing room for another three months.

"A perinatologist came in to see me. After giving me a physical exam and a sonogram, he found that the placenta was covering my cervix and a clot behind the placenta was forcing it to separate from the uterine wall (he called it placenta previa and abruption). Once the doctors knew why I was bleeding they went into action to try to stop a premature delivery. First they put me in a Trendelenburg bed that elevated my hips and feet. This was done in an effort to counter the pull of gravity on the baby. (It amazed me that in this age of advanced medical technology, the first method of forestalling premature birth was to hang me upside down!) My obstetrician suggested that I try to make myself comfortable in that position because she hoped I would be able to hold on to the baby for at least another six weeks. (She wanted me to lie upside down for six weeks?!) As awful as this seemed, I was willing to try anything.

"After only a few hours, the doctors realized that the Trendelenburg bed wasn't enough; the contractions were getting stronger. Now, instead of hoping to hold off delivery for six weeks, they hoped only for forty-eight hours—just long enough to give a drug called betamethasone a chance to speed up the development of the baby's lungs. I hadn't taken any medication, not even an aspirin, during my pregnancy, and like my first delivery, I planned to have a totally natural childbirth. I wanted my obstetrician to find some way to get me through this without any drugs, but this time she convinced me that betamethasone, along with a tocolytic agent called Brethine (which would slow down the contractions), were my only hope of holding my baby in the uterus, where every additional hour improved his chances of survival. So there I was—someone who had planned to do everything naturally—lying upside down, strapped to monitors, with an IV in my arm, and with drugs running through my body, praying double-time that my baby would be okay.

"My obstetrician, who had always been supportive, didn't offer any encouragement now. She kept shaking her head, saying, 'It's just too soon.' But my obstetrician didn't know my Stephanie. She was born (just fifteen hours after I was admitted to the hospital) kicking, crying, and letting everyone in the birthing room know that she was here to stay."

In the future, medical scientists may find more exact reasons for premature labor, and better, more effective ways to stop it. But for now, the simple fact is: Sometimes babies are born early. Fortunately, medical science has advanced to the point where, like little Stephanie, the majority of babies born after the twenty-fifth week of gestation will grow to be normal, healthy children.

Even though this is encouraging information, when your preemie is born, you'll probably want to know how he is different from a full-term baby, why he needs special care, and how long it will be before he's "full grown." The chart of fetal development printed below will help you start to answer these questions. Find your premature baby's gestational birth age on this chart. Then, looking over the weeks before his birth, you'll be able to see how much he had already developed in utero. By reading ahead on the chart, you'll see how much more he needs to grow out of utero before he can be compared to a full-term baby.

Before you do this, you should know that a discussion of fetal age can be a bit confusing and warrants some explanation. The lunar method of calculating a baby's age at birth is in standard use throughout the fields of obstetrics and neonatology, and will be used throughout this book. This method measures a full-term pregnancy in ten lunar months, or 40 weeks. Therefore, if a baby is born 10 weeks prematurely, he is said to be 30 gestational weeks old. However, when discussing premature birth, in which every day since conception is counted so carefully, trying to calculate your baby's exact age can be somewhat confusing. This is because the 40-week pregnancy is counted from the first day of the mother's last menstrual period, although most often the baby is not conceived until at least two weeks later. So when a baby is described as being 30 gestational weeks old, he has probably really been in existence for only 28 weeks. What all this means is: Your baby's exact age is difficult to determine because ovulation and conception can occur at any time during that two-week period after the onset of menstruation. For this reason, when examining the beginnings of embryonic development on the chart below, the first signs of growth begin at week 2.

Fetal Development

Gestational Age	Fetal Development
Weeks 1 and 2	Menstruation and ovulation.
Weeks 3 to 4	Fertilization, cell division, implantation of the embryo in the uterus.
Week 5	The head and the tail folds are distinct. The primary brain vesicles form. The nervous system begins to develop. The optic vesicles and lens form. Limb buds are present. The earliest form of the liver, pancreas, lungs, thyroid gland, and heart appear. Two heart tubes are fused in the midline and begin to contract.
Week 6	The embryo is curled in a C shape. The head, tail, and arm buds are easily recognizable. The arm buds have divided into hand, arm, and shoulder units. The leg buds have divided into thigh, leg, and foot units. The heart bulges from the body. The cerebral brain hemispheres are enlarging. In the stomach area, the primary intestinal loop is present. On the face, the nostrils have overhanging borders. The eyes appear as dark spots.

Week 7   The fetus weighs $1/1,000$ of an ounce.
The head is relatively larger.
The trunk of the main body is elongating and straightening.
On the head, the ears and nostrils are continuing to develop shape.
The tip of the nose is present.
The eyelid folds are forming.
Finger and toe digits are evident.
The elbows are present.
In the heart, there is complete separation between the right and left atrioventricular canal; the aortic and pulmonary valves are distinct.
In the mid-area, the appendix and pancreas are present, and the midgut herniates into the umbilical cord.
The secondary bronchi of the lungs are branched.
The arms are longer and begin to bend at the elbows and and curve slightly over the heart.
The pituitary gland is forming in the middle of the brain.
Spleen and liver ducts are forming.
The intestines elongate.
The cerebral cortex (the part of the brain that directs motor activity and intellect) can be seen.
The stomach and esophagus begin to form.
Muscles appear in the pelvic region.

Week 8   The fetus is $1/2$ inch long.
The heart is beating 65 times per minute.
The hands are flexed over the wrists and meet over the heart bulge.

The fingers are longer and the tips are slightly swollen where touch pads are developing.

The feet are approaching the midline and may meet.

The eyelids have almost covered the eyes.

The external ear is well advanced in form.

The head is in a more erect position and the neck is more developed.

The limbs are longer.

Cartilage appears where bones will later develop.

The head is bent forward onto the chest.

The eyes develop pigment.

The mouth may open for the first time.

The jaws are well formed.

Nerve fibers connect the olfactory lobe of the brain, laying the groundwork for the sense of smell.

The brain stem is now recognizable.

Lung buds can be seen.

Week 9   Using ultrasound, the first fetal movements can be detected.

The nerve cells of the eyes' retinas form.

The semicircular canals of the ears form.

The nasal passages open to the outside.

The tongue forms from the floor of the mouth.

The nerve connections from the retina to the brain are established.

A distinct neck connects the head to the body.

All fingers are present.

The urological and rectal passages are completely separate.

Week 10   The fetus now weighs $\frac{1}{13}$ of an ounce and is $1\frac{1}{4}$ inches from the top of the head to the rump.
The eyes have moved from the sides of the head closer to the front.
Bones begin to replace the cartilage.
The stomach moves into its final position.
Taste buds begin to form.
Neck muscles are forming.
The clitoris appears in the female and the ovaries begin to descend.
The testes begin to descend within the body of the male.
The two lobes of the lungs extend into many tiny tubes (bronchioles).
The diaphragm begins to separate the heart and lungs from the stomach.
Muscles are sufficiently developed to allow movement.
At the end of week 10, the embryonic period is complete and the fetal period begins. This period is characterized by the rapid growth of the fetus and the further differentiation of the organs and tissues formed in the embryonic period.

Week 11   The head is almost half the size of the fetus.
The eyelids have fused together and will stay that way until week 24.
The fingernails appear.
The external genitalia are developing.
The hair follicles of the skin are forming.
The ears are still abnormally low on the sides of the head.
Teeth are beginning to form.

Week 12   The fetus weighs $\frac{1}{4}$ of an ounce and is about $2\frac{1}{3}$ inches long.

A skeleton of cartilage is forming.
The gallbladder secretes bile from the fetus.
The lungs are completely formed.
The palate (the upper part of the mouth) is formed.
The thyroid gland and pancreas are now complete.
If the forehead is touched, the fetus will turn its head away.

Week 13   The fetus is about 3 inches long (double its length at week 7).
The beginnings of finger- and footprints begin to form.
Tooth buds appear for all 20 baby teeth.
The vocal cords begin to form.
The trachea, lungs, stomach, liver, pancreas, and intestines are developed into their final functioning form.

Week 14   The ears have moved from the neck onto the head.
The eyes have moved to the front of the face.
The genitalia have fully differentiated into male or female.
The digestive glands are complete.
The taste buds are numerous and the salivary glands form.
The vocal cords are complete.

Week 15   The skin is very thin and the blood vessels can easily be seen through this translucent covering.

Week 16   The fetus can make a fist, open its mouth, move its lips, and swallow.
The fetus may suck its thumb.
Fine lanugo hairs can be seen on the head.

The nails are well formed.
The legs are longer than the arms.
The heart is beating 117 to 157 times per minute.
The stomach is producing digestive juices.
The liver is making blood cells.
The kidneys are producing urine.

Week 17
Brown fat begins to form.
The period of rapid growth rate begins to slow down.
A white fatty material begins to enclose the nerve fibers of the spinal cord.
Between the seventeenth and twentieth weeks the hearing develops; the fetus can hear internal-organ and outside-world sounds.

Week 18
The skeleton is clearly outlined on X-rays of the fetus.
Lanugo covers the entire body.

Week 19
The fetus is about 5²/₃ inches long.
Parts of the leg reach their relative proportion.
The mother can feel active fetal movements as the fetus kicks, moves its arms, and wiggles its fingers and toes.

Week 20
A skin covering called vernix caseosa forms to protect the skin from the amniotic fluid.

Week 21
Body parts, tissues, and organs continue to mature.

Week 22
The eyelids are very well developed.
Fingernails are completely developed.

Weeks 23 to 27	The body is beginning to become plump. The lanugo darkens. The skin becomes wrinkled. The face and the body generally assume the appearance of an infant at birth. The eyes are open again. Fetuses born from week 25 onward are usually capable of sustaining life.
Weeks 28 to 31	The eyebrows and eyelashes are well developed. The scalp hairs are growing.
Weeks 32 to 36	The body is becoming plumper. Toenails are present. Fingernails have reached the tips of the fingers.
Weeks 37 to 40	The body is fully plump. The toenails have reached the tips of the toes. Almost all the lanugo hair is gone. The testes have descended into the scrotum, but the ovaries are still above the level of the pelvic bone and will not reach their full position by birth. The fetus gains approximately half a pound each week.

Chapter Two

. . . .

Routine Medical Care for a Preemie

SPECIAL PROCEDURES

Peggy and Bob's son, Jason, was born prematurely. Peggy sometimes thinks back to the time during her pregnancy when she daydreamed about what it would be like right after she gave birth. "I imagined that Bob and I would be smiling through teary eyes, as we cuddled with our newborn for the first time and waved to the home video camera. Well, I found out right away that if your baby comes early, it's just not like that. I gave one last hard push; my obstetrician said, 'It's a boy,' and then a swarm of people whisked my baby away. I stared up at the bright lights on the ceiling and started to cry. This wasn't how I imagined it was supposed to be. My husband and my baby were both gone and all that was left for me were questions—hundreds of questions, such as: 'Where did they take my baby?' 'Who are all those people?' 'What are they doing to him?' 'Is he all right?' 'When can I see him?' I was sure I'd go crazy if one more person said, 'We're doing everything we can.' I needed to know more."

Peggy's delivery room experience is a typical one for

many women who deliver a premature infant. No one involved in your baby's birth intends to ignore you, or minimize your fears and concerns, but your baby's health
comes first. Since every moment without treatment can be
dangerous for a preemie, many of your initial questions
may go unanswered. When it is finally time to visit your
baby and ask your questions, your ability to concentrate
on the facts may be clouded by the excitement of the moment, and by the wires and tubes and monitors that appear
to overwhelm your tiny newborn. And so you will still have
unanswered questions.

This chapter will answer the kinds of questions most
commonly asked by parents in the first few days after the
birth of their premature baby—questions about the medical
equipment and procedures being used, about the hospital
facilities, and about the seeming "swarms" of people involved in the care of their child. Although the exact type
and sequence of medical care will depend on individual
hospital and doctor policy, as well as on the gestational age
and birth weight of each baby (as explained in Chapters
Four, Five, and Six), there are some procedures and medical specialists that are routinely a part of caring for preemies.

What's Happening to My Baby?

When Jason was "whisked" away from Peggy and Bob, his
doctors began a series of procedures that would determine
future treatment, and that would help him adapt to the environment outside his mother's uterus. Immediately after
birth, a preemie is placed on a radiant warmer, which is a
small open bed with a heat source overhead. Because a
preemie is born with very little body fat to help regulate
his body temperature, and with too little muscle strength
to generate heat by shivering, his body temperature is ar-

tificially regulated on this warmer. At the same time that the preemie needs heat, doctors and nurses need complete visual and physical access to a fully exposed baby. Because the radiant warmer gives both warmth and easy access, it is an essential piece of equipment. Once on the warmer, your baby will be carefully and completely dried with warmed towels to further reduce heat loss.

When the baby is one minute of age, the doctor will determine an Apgar score to evaluate how well he is adapting to the outside world. This rating system is named after its originator, Dr. Virginia Apgar. Her name is now used as an acronym for five areas of evaluation:

A: appearance (especially skin color)

P: pulse rate (number of heart beats per minute)

G: grimace (a baby's response to annoying stimulation, such as a tap or a finger flick to the body)

A: activity (muscle tone is tested through observation and by flexing and feeling the tension in the baby's arms and legs)

R: respiration (how well the baby can breathe and cry on his own)

A combined Apgar score under seven indicates that the baby is in some kind of distress and needs medical treatment. This evaluation is administered again at five and ten minutes of age so the doctors can follow the baby's progress or deterioration.

Jason's first Apgar score read like this:

Appearance	0
Pulse	2
Grimace	1
Activity	1
Respiration	1
Combined	$\overline{5}$

Each of these factors is rated on a scale of 0 to 2 with 2 being the most desirable score, thereby making 10 a perfect score. These numbers are determined by the following criteria:

Sign	0	1	2
Appearance	blue or pale	body pink: extremities blue	completely pink
Pulse Rate	absent	slow (less than 100 beats per minute)	greater than 100 beats per minute
Grimace	no response	grimace	cough or sneeze
Activity	limp	some flexion	active motion
Respiration	absent	weak cry	good, strong cry

Source: Adapted from Apgar Score Chart, *Journal of the American Medical Association,* Vol. 168, No. 15, p. 1985. Copyright 1985, American Medical Association. Reprinted with permission.

These numbers alerted Jason's doctors to his need for oxygen, stimulation, warmth, and further observation.

Five minutes later, Jason's second Apgar score read like this:

Appearance	1
Pulse	2
Grimace	2
Activity	1
Respiration	2
Combined	8

This change for the better indicated that the doctors' efforts to stabilize Jason's vital signs were proving successful. Between Apgar evaluations the doctors and nurses used medical procedures that helped improve the baby's scores. Because Jason's color was blue-grey and his breathing was shallow and labored at birth, they immediately suctioned his mouth to remove excess mucus and blood, and then gave him humidified oxygen. (Doctors will promptly give resuscitative assistance to any baby who is not breathing spontaneously and/or whose heart rate is less than 80 to 100 beats per minute.)

Also between Apgar evaluations, the medical personnel perform the procedures for routine newborn care. They draw a tube of blood from the placental umbilical cord, which is used to identify the baby's blood type and Rh group. Then they place an identification band around his wrist or ankle. This band states the mother's admission number, the baby's sex, and the date and time of birth. The baby is then footprinted, and the mother is fingerprinted. Although some hospitals are now using new blood typing techniques for this identification, the foot- and fingerprinting routine is still common, and a copy of the baby's footprint is often given to the parents as a keepsake.

This initial series of evaluative and stabilizing procedures is done right in the delivery room, and usually takes only a few minutes. If time and conditions allow, most doctors give the parents a chance to see their baby just before he leaves the delivery room. Then the preemie is wrapped in warmed thermal blankets, placed in a movable, temperature-controlled incubator, and transferred to the nursery where his care will continue.

Bob was allowed to follow Jason into the nursery, but Peggy would have only a quick glimpse of Jason to last her the next twenty-four hours. "The doctor folded down the flap of a blanket," remembers Peggy, "and let me have a fast look. This at least gave me a picture to hold in my mind. It was my only concrete proof that I did have a baby. It sounds silly, but that one-second peek gave me a lot of comfort until I could finally see Jason again.''

In the nursery, your preemie is again placed on a radiant warmer to maintain his body temperature while the doctors and nurses continue to examine and evaluate his condition. Within the first few hours in the nursery, your baby will receive a full physical exam, his weight, length, and head circumference will be measured, X-rays (if necessary) will be taken, urine and feces will be collected for analysis, and blood samples (usually taken from a vein or an artery or from the baby's heel) will be drawn to gather information such as oxygen, carbon dioxide, sodium, and sugar levels. All of this data will be used to evaluate the condition of the baby after birth and to determine how to care for him in the immediate future.

What Are All Those Wires?

When you go to visit your new baby, he'll probably be hooked up to what look like a bunch of wires. These are monitoring wires and although they can be frightening, even intimidating at first, they aren't doing anything *to* your baby. They are taking vital information *from* your baby and allowing his doctors and nurses to watch his progress closely every second of the night and day without ever pricking, sticking, jabbing, or in any other way hurting the preemie.

There will most likely be at least five wires running from small electrodes (sensors that are secured to your baby's skin) back to electronic read-out monitors. (See illustration, page 45). These wires and monitors allow the doctors and nurses to evaluate and oversee the following four functions that are prime indicators of stability:

1. Body Temperature

It is very important for a preemie to have a stabilized body temperature. As explained earlier, because a preemie doesn't have enough body fat to keep his body temperature at an acceptable level, he is warmed by external heating units. These units are adjusted to provide just enough warmth to keep the air surrounding the baby at between 32 and 37 degrees centigrade (89.6°–98.6° fahrenheit).

In addition to monitoring the air around the baby, the baby's skin temperature is recorded by a monitoring sensor that is usually attached to his abdomen. Generally, if his temperature goes below 98°, he is in danger of losing oxygen and weight, and of having a dangerous buildup of lactic acid in the body. If the body temperature goes above 99.5°, it is likely that his skin will flush, his heart rate will increase, he may experience breathing pauses, and he may suffer weight loss. If his body temperature goes above or below the range his doctor feels best for him, the monitor will detect the change and automatically regulate the surrounding air temperature, or an alarm will sound.

2. Oxygen Levels

For a human being to survive, there must be a certain amount of oxygen in the blood. The preemie's level of oxygen can be measured with a heat- or light-activated sensor. Both have advantages and disadvantages.

A heat-activated sensor may measure partial pressure of oxygen, as well as partial pressure of carbon dioxide. Using this kind of monitor, the doctors can make sure that your baby's oxygen level remains over the range of 50 to 60 mm of mercury, and the carbon dioxide level stays under the range of 40 to 50 mm of mercury. This dual reading from one sensor is a convenient and noninvasive way to get information that is necessary for the complete and ongoing evaluation of your baby. But it has one drawback: It is possible that the baby's fragile skin may be burned because, to get an accurate reading, heat must be used to warm the skin.

A light-activated sensor uses a pulse oximeter to measure the amount of oxygen bound to the hemoglobin molecules in the blood (called the oxygen saturation level). This monitor often has an individualized preset alarm limit that alerts the nurses when the oxygen level falls below the amount appropriate for each baby. But, generally, if a preemie's oxygen saturation level falls below the range of 85 to 90 breaths per minute, an alarm will sound. Although this kind of light-activated sensor gives a clear recording of the levels of oxygen getting into the baby's system, and it does it in a noninvasive way and without burning the baby's skin, it does not measure the level of carbon dioxide in the blood. If your baby's oxygen level is being monitored with a pulse oximeter, his carbon dioxide level will be checked by drawing blood samples for laboratory analysis.

3. Heart and Breathing Rates

Three wires connected to a single monitor are usually used to measure heart and breathing rates. One sensor attached to your baby's chest will record the baby's heart rate by measuring the electrical output of the heart. An acceptable heart rate for a preemie falls between 110 and 160 beats per minute. (The average adult heart rate is between 60 and 80 beats per minute.) A second wire, usually attached to your baby's chest or abdomen, measures the stretching movement of the chest and/or abdomen and records the baby's rate of respiration. This breathing rate should not fall below 30 breaths per minute. The third wire, usually attached to a lower extremity, acts as a ground wire, which is needed to prevent electrical interference. These three wires meet in the lead box and their signals are transmitted and displayed on the monitor. (See illustration, page 45.)

The alarm on this monitor will sound for a number of reasons: It will ring if your baby stops breathing (a condition called apnea). It will also ring if the baby's heartbeat and/or respiration rate go above or below preset levels. For example, a physician may set the alarm to ring if the baby's heart rate falls below 100 beats per minute (a condition called bradycardia), or above 200 beats per minute, or if his respiration rate goes too high (usually above 80 breaths per minute).

If the alarm does go off—don't panic. About 45 percent of babies weighing less than 5 pounds, and 85 percent of those under 2 pounds have apnea episodes during the first few weeks of life; these are often accompanied by a bout of bradycardia. Most preemies grow out of apnea by the time they reach 34 to 35 weeks postconceptual age, but a few will continue to experience these episodes for weeks, or even months longer. If your baby continues to experience these breathing pauses when he's otherwise ready to go home, his doctors may prescribe medications that improve respiration, or they may order an apnea monitor for you to use at home.

Peggy and Bob both remember the first time the alarm rang on Jason's respiratory monitor. "It happened on the first day that I went to see him in the nursery," recalls Peggy. "I was nervous to begin with, and I was trying so hard to remember all the things the nurse was telling me. All of a sudden, this awful shrill sound started screaming from one of the monitors and a red light was flashing. I thought Jason was in some kind of terrible trouble and I felt so helpless because I couldn't do anything for him. But none of the nurses seemed at all upset. I remember, I grabbed one of them and started yelling at her to do something to help my baby. I guess I expected her to call in some kind of medical SWAT team, but instead she just tapped the bottom of his foot a few times. The alarm and the light stopped, and I had my first embarrassing lesson in how to handle a mild episode of apnea."

Many preemies have irregular breathing patterns. They

may take several short breaths, stop breathing for ten seconds or so, and then resume a normal breathing rate. This kind of breathing pattern (called periodic breathing) may cause the respiratory alarm to sound, but it does not affect the baby's color, muscle tone, or heart rate, and it is not a cause for concern. If, however, the pause lasts for more than 15 to 20 seconds, the baby is having an apnea spell; this can usually be remedied with gentle stimulation, such as rubbing or tapping his arm or leg. To prevent breathing pauses, your baby may be placed on a constant-motion waterbed mattress or on one with a rocking device that continuously and gently reminds him to breathe.

Sometimes a preemie may have a severe or extended apnea spell. This can cause the baby to turn a blue-grey color as his oxygen level begins to drop, or a pale color if the oxygen is redirected away from the skin to the most important internal organs. If the baby doesn't respond to gentle stimulation, he will be given forced air (sometimes with added oxygen) through a bag and mask that fits over his nose and mouth. If apnea pauses occur more than five to ten times a day, he may be given medication (such as caffeine or theophylline) to encourage a regular breathing pattern, or the baby may be put on a respirator and checked for an underlying cause such as low levels of blood sugar or calcium, infection, or a disorder of the central nervous system.

The respiratory and heart rate monitor is an invaluable piece of equipment in the care of premature babies, but the sound of its alarm has probably caused more parental anxiety than it has alerted anyone to real infant distress. This is especially true when the monitor rings out a false alarm, which can easily happen if one of the wires gets twisted, kinked, or dislodged, or if a sensor loosens, or if the baby's movements interfere with accurate readings. When you're in the nursery, use the monitor alarms as a signal to look at your baby. If his color and breathing pattern are unchanged, there's no need to panic. A nurse will also come by quickly to observe the baby, reassure you, reset the monitor, and/or intervene if necessary.

For the rest of your baby's stay in the preemie nursery, the doctors and nurses will use the body temperature, oxygen level, and heart and breathing rate monitors to be sure your baby's condition remains stable.

On his first day in the nursery, Jason's monitors looked like this:

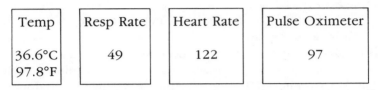

Temp	Resp Rate	Heart Rate	Pulse Oximeter
36.6°C 97.8°F	49	122	97

At a glance, these numbers told the doctors and nurses that Jason was doing fine. If, however, the initial medical exam and/or monitor readings should indicate that your baby has a medical problem requiring intervention, the doctors will explain the problem to you, decide on a course of action, and ask for your permission to proceed. If the problem is severe enough to call for highly specialized personnel and facilities, your baby may be transferred to another hospital. (See page 47 for a full discussion of hospital facilities.)

What Are All Those Tubes?

Respiratory Equipment

Like many other preemies, Jason had difficulty breathing when he was first born. Although his lungs were completely formed, they didn't have enough of a chemical called surfactant, which helps expand the small air sacs in the lungs. This condition, called respiratory distress syndrome (RDS) or hyaline membrane disease (HMD), can usually be controlled by one of the following three procedures until the baby matures and begins to produce surfactant on his own.

1. Oxygen Hood

Babies with the mildest degree of RDS (or a mild degree of cardiac illness, or infection) will usually have an oxygen hood placed over their heads. This is a clear plastic box into which air with varying amounts of added oxygen is pumped through a tube.

The air inside the oxygen hood may also contain warmed moisture. This is added to make sure the secretions and tissues of the baby's airways and lungs do not dry out, and also to help loosen the mucus that the baby cannot cough out of his lungs. (This mucus will be periodically suctioned out.) The moisture may fog up the hood, making it seem as if the baby is in grave distress, but actually it's normal, expected, and an inconsequential side effect of warm air being pushed against the cooler plastic walls of the hood.

While a baby is under the hood, the levels of oxygen he receives will be carefully controlled and monitored. The levels will be gradually diminished until he is able to breathe room air (which is 21 percent oxygen) on his own without any difficulty or risk of complication.

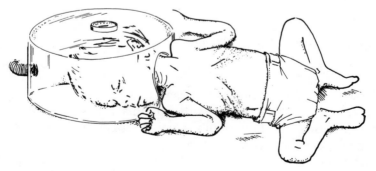

Oxygen Hood

2. Continuous Positive Airway Pressure

Some babies can breathe on their own most of the time, but occasionally may need some help getting air into their lungs. In this case, instead of the oxygen hood, a tube that provides a constant flow of air will be placed into one (or both) nostrils. This continuous positive airway pressure (CPAP) will force air through the pharynx, vocal cords, and trachea, and then into the lungs. (This procedure may also be called positive end expiratory pressure or PEEP.) Like the oxygen hood, this air is humidified (added moisture) and supplemental oxygen is added as needed. With newer applications and earlier use of CPAP doctors are now able, in some cases, to avoid the use of the respirator (see #3, "Respiratory Intubation"), and thereby decrease the occurrence of complications such as chronic lung disease, oxygen dependency, and the need for intubation (placement of a tube through the vocal cords into the trachea).

As the baby shows signs of being able to get air into his lungs on his own, he will be slowly weaned from CPAP to the oxygen hood.

3. Endotracheal Intubation

Babies with the most severe degree of RDS may need actual breathing assistance. In this case, an air tube is

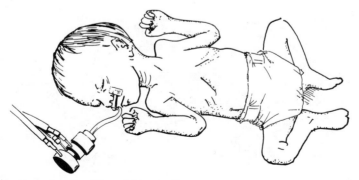

Continuous Positive Airway Pressure

threaded through the baby's nose or mouth, down the back of his throat, and into the trachea (windpipe). This tube is connected to a respirator that regulates the flow of air, oxygen, and air pressure as they go in and out of the lungs. Most commonly, this kind of respiration is given by way of intermittent mandatory ventilation (IMV).

Although sometimes IMV respiration does all the breathing for the baby, most commonly the respirations given by IMV are done in a pattern that is harmonious with the baby's own breathing rate. For example, if the respirator is set to "breathe" 20 times per minute (once every 3 seconds), the baby may breathe on his own once or twice in between each forced-air breath of the IMV. Sometimes, however, IMV respiration must do all the breathing for the baby. In these cases the baby may be sedated to prevent him from fighting or working against the respirator.

Of these three respiratory aids, IMV carries the greatest risk of complication. The constant pressure of forced air may cause a preemie's lungs to pop, or it may traumatize the airways of the lungs and cause chronic lung disease. (See Chapter Three for a full discussion of bronchopulmonary dysplasia.) If your baby's doctors have decided to use this procedure, it is because, their first priority, like yours, is to keep your baby breathing and alive.

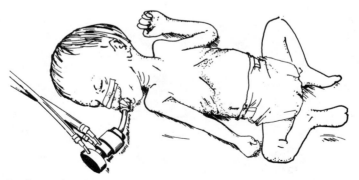

Endotracheal Tube

All respiratory management procedures are closely monitored by doctors, nurses, and respiratory therapists. The amount of added oxygen may range from 21 to 100 percent; the monitors assure the doctors that the amount being given to the baby is, in fact, what he needs. As the baby's lungs improve, the level of oxygen and the rate of forced air will be steadily decreased until he is completely weaned off the supplemental oxygen supply. Most preemies are ready to breathe on their own within the first week after birth.

It's interesting to note that initial respiratory distress is eight to ten times greater in babies born by scheduled and/ or elective cesarean deliveries. This sometimes happens because C-section babies do not have the benefit of the uterine contractions that push on their thorax and rid them of the excess fluid that collects in the chest cavity. The resulting respiratory problems usually improve after twelve to twenty-four hours on IV fluids and respiratory support systems.

Methods of Feeding

• **Intravenous Feeding:** To grow in size and strength, your baby needs nutrients and calories. How these are given depends on the preemie's individual needs. Because most preemies have an immature digestive tract that isn't ready to take in food, your baby probably will be nourished initially through intravenous (IV) lines that carry a solution directly into his bloodstream. Initially, the solution contains only carbohydrates (sugar), and electrolytes (sodium and potassium). Gradually, protein, minerals, vitamins, and then fat are added to provide a solution called total parenteral nutrition. This method of feeding is most often used with preemies younger than 34 weeks gestational age, who can not yet suck, swallow, and breathe in a coordinated manner, and/or with those who are being treated for other health complications, such as infection or respiratory distress syndrome.

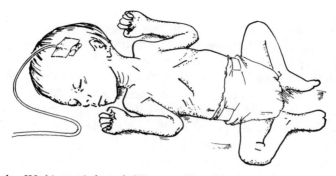

Scalp IV (A peripheral IV may also be inserted into a vein located in the arm or leg.)

Depending on your baby's needs, his doctor will choose one of the following four methods to begin his intake of parenteral nutrition:

1. Peripheral Intravenous

The safest intravenous feeding route is through a peripheral vein (one close to the skin's surface). For this kind of IV feeding, a very small needle or plastic catheter is inserted into a vein in the baby's arm, leg, or scalp. If the IV is inserted into an arm or leg, it may be secured by a splint and wrapped with gauze so the baby can't easily dislodge it when he moves. Very often a scalp vein will be used because there are numerous veins on the head that are close to the surface and easy to locate, and also because the baby will be less likely to dislodge the needle. You might feel uneasy seeing your baby with a scalp IV because his hair will be shaved at the point of insertion, and the needle might look to you as if it were going directly into the brain, but relax—your baby's hair will all grow back, the veins of the scalp are in no way connected to the brain, and the procedure is appropriate, quite safe, and relatively painless.

Peripheral IVs are the safest way to administer parenteral nutrients, but solutions with high concentrations of sugar cannot be given for a long period of time without risking infection or vein inflammation. To avoid this problem, your baby's IV will be moved to new locations every twenty-four to forty-eight hours. One day he may be feeding through an IV in his scalp and the next day it will be moved down to his arm or leg. When an IV line is removed, you might notice a bruise on the skin at the point where the needle went in. This often happens, even to adults, and is generally not a cause for concern. But sometimes, if too much fluid passes through the tube, or if the needle dislodges from the vein, fluid may seep out into the surrounding tissues and the child may then show signs of a skin burn and suffer permanent scarring. The possibility of this happening, however, is greatly reduced by careful wrapping and securing of the IV (that's why you'll see lots of tape holding the needle in place), and by the infusion pump attached to the IV line that carefully regulates in precisely measured amounts the fluids going into your baby's bloodstream. The nurses will also check the insertion site frequently and change it when necessary.

2. Umbilical Catheter

During the first or second day of life, your preemie may be given parenteral nutrition through an umbilical catheter. This is a tube that is surgically placed into a vessel (usually the vein) of the baby's umbilical cord (belly button). Since there are no nerves in the umbilical cord, this procedure is entirely painless. An umbilical catheter may also be threaded through the umbilical artery directly into the baby's aorta (the large artery leading away from the heart). This kind of umbilical artery catheter (called a UAC or UA line) may also be used to deliver nutrition, but most often it is used to monitor blood pressure and to draw blood for analysis.

In some circumstances, an umbilical catheter is the best way to feed a preemie. Because it is inserted into a large blood vessel, a catheter can deliver high concentrations of nutrients without fear of burning surrounding tissues. Be-

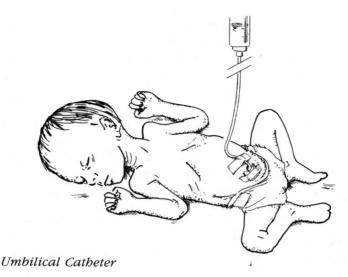

Umbilical Catheter

cause it is surgically implanted, it can remain in place for several days without becoming dislodged.

However, despite the convenience, an umbilical catheter carries more potential risks (such as infection and/or blood clots) than the other intravenous feeding methods. Therefore, it is generally used only with the most critically ill infants and with those who may need intravenous feedings for several weeks. For these babies, umbilical catheters are the safest, most appropriate way to continually supply fluids and food to the body and draw out the needed blood samples.

3. A "Cut Down"

A third way to deliver parenteral nutrition to your baby is through an IV tube inserted into a larger vein of the arm or leg and then threaded through that vein to a large blood vessel near the heart. This tube is sometimes inserted with a needle that is withdrawn when the tube is in place, or by a minor surgical procedure called a "cut down." In this case, either a neonatologist or a pediatric surgeon will anesthetize the area, then make an incision over the vein and put the IV tube in place.

There are advantages as well as drawbacks to using this technique. It is used instead of a peripheral IV when the doctors can no longer find suitable peripheral veins. It can give the baby a higher concentration of nutrients than can be administered safely through a surface vein, and it can be used when the doctor expects the baby to need intravenous feedings for several weeks. Although this kind of tube feeding eliminates the risks involved when a peripheral IV becomes dislodged or allows fluids to seep into surrounding tissues, it increases the risk of infection by placing a foreign object (the tube) so far into the baby's body. If your baby is feeding through this kind of IV tube, he will be closely monitored for any sign of infection. If an infection should develop, the tube will probably be removed immediately.

4. Broviac Catheter

When it is expected that a preemie will not be able to tolerate oral feedings for an exceptionally long period of time (weeks, months, or even years) his doctors may choose to deliver his nutrients and fluids through a broviac catheter. This catheter is threaded through a large vein in the baby's neck, and (unlike other catheters) it has a separate exit site through the skin over the chest wall. Because placement of the broviac catheter is an intricate surgical procedure, it is done under anesthesia in the operating room. (In certain circumstances local anesthesia may be used.)

Like the IV tube inserted with a cut-down procedure, the advantage of a broviac catheter is that it can be used for extended periods of time; it does not become dislodged, nor does it allow fluids to seep into surrounding tissues. However, it increases the risk of infection, and because it is surgically placed with the use of anesthesia, it

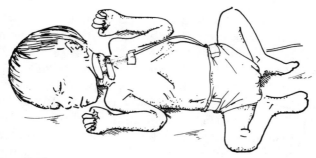

Broviac Catheter

is used only when absolutely necessary and with careful monitoring of the baby's vital signs.

• **Oral Feedings**: After intravenous feedings are established, oral feedings will gradually be introduced as your baby is able to digest breast milk or formula, and as he shows signs of growing strength and stability. Although your baby's digestive system may be ready for breast milk or formula, his coordinated ability to suck, swallow, and breathe may not yet be developed. That's why most preemies begin oral feedings through a narrow flexible tube threaded through their nose or mouth, down the esophagus, and directly into the stomach. If the tube is threaded through the nose, it is called a naso-gastric tube (NG tube); if it is threaded through the mouth, it is called an oro-gastric tube. Sometimes this kind of feeding is also called a gavage feeding. Most often the NG tube is left in place to administer intermittent feedings as needed. Since most preemies haven't developed the gag reflex yet, they don't seem to mind. If, however, the tube causes the baby any distress, it can be withdrawn after each feeding and reinserted when needed again.

These oral feedings are often begun while the preemie is still getting intravenous feedings. At first the NG tube will be used to give the baby a small amount of sugar water. If

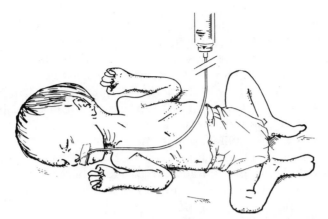

Naso-Gastric Tube (If the tube is threaded through the baby's mouth, it is called an oro-gastric tube.)

his digestive tract can tolerate this, he may be given small amounts of half-strength or full-strength breast milk or formula. Then if all continues to go well, the IV feedings will be gradually diminished while the NG tube feedings are continually increased. Eventually the NG tube alone will be used to feed your baby from ½ to 1 ounce of milk every 2 to 3 hours.

Peggy was delighted when Jason graduated to the NG tube. "It was the first time since his birth that I felt like I had some control over his treatment and health. I had been pumping, freezing, and storing my breast milk because I had read that breast milk is especially nourishing to preemies." (She's right! Human milk contains anti-infectious factors and it aids in the digestion of fats by supplementing the baby's short supply of pancreatic lipase.) "Although Jason still needed a formula fortified with protein, calcium, and phosphorus, he was also getting MY milk. Finally, I was able to give my baby something that no one else could give him, and it made me feel great!"

Naso-gastric feedings can also give your preemie a chance to practice his sucking and maybe even jump ahead in growth. Recent studies have found that preemies who are allowed to suck on a pacifier during tube feedings often require fewer days of these feedings than those who do not suck. Some also gain more weight, have fewer complications, and are released from the hospital sooner. If your baby is being fed with an NG tube, ask your doctor about this kind of nonnutritive sucking.

Most preemies will stay with the NG tube until their condition is stable. This status is reached when (1) the baby is no longer getting respirator or oxygen therapy, (2) he is gaining weight; and (3) he can coordinate the sucking, swallowing, and breathing reflex. This usually comes together when the baby is about 34 weeks postconceptual age. Then your baby will graduate to feeding from a bottle with a specially designed nipple that encourages him to suck for his food, yet won't make him too tired. Once he is used to sucking while eating, his health is stable, and he is about four pounds, you can begin to breast-feed him if you choose.

Waiting for your baby to grow so you can hold him in your arms and feed him can be very difficult as each day crawls into the next without any observable signs of change. But each day your baby is growing stronger. If you are patient and remember the one-day-at-a-time approach to caring for him, he'll be in your arms sucking contentedly on the bottle or breast before you know it.

Before concluding this section on feeding methods, it seems appropriate to mention that after your baby is born he will lose up to 10 percent of his total body weight no matter which feeding method is used. This happens (even to full-term babies) because, in the first few days, babies cannot feed well enough, or take in enough nutrients to match the amount of fluids and nutrients they had been receiving from the placenta. It usually takes one to three weeks before the baby will get back up to his birth

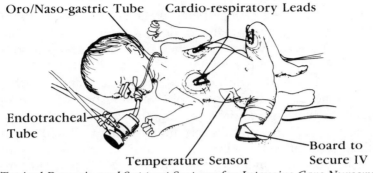

Oro/Naso-gastric Tube   Cardio-respiratory Leads

Endotracheal Tube

Temperature Sensor   Board to Secure IV

Typical Preemie and Support Systems for Intensive Care Nursery

weight. (The smaller the baby the longer it takes.) When you hear that your baby is losing weight—don't worry that something is wrong with him or with the way he is being fed. This initial weight loss is not a step backward; it is a normal and expected step forward on the road to recovery.

The illustration above shows you the kind of equipment that is generally used to monitor, stabilize, and support the vital signs of premature infants. Although your baby may be hooked up a bit differently, this picture will still help to answer the question, "What are all those wires and tubes?"

When your baby's health is stable and he is in no imminent danger (this assessment can take from one hour to several days to make), he will be transferred from the radiant warmer to an incubator. This is an enclosed, see-through, temperature-controlled, sometimes double-walled, box. An incubator gives a preemie environmental protection from germs and drafts. It has portholelike doors that allow doctors, nurses, and you to make contact with the baby without taking him out of his sheltered home.

Although your baby will come out of his incubator each

day to be bathed, changed, and weighed, until he is about 34 weeks postconceptual age (or four pounds) the incubator is where you will watch him day by day as he grows in size, strength, and personality.

The first day that Bob entered the nursery and saw that Jason had been moved from his warming bed to an incubator he became frantic. "I thought that because the incubator looks more cumbersome and is totally enclosed, Jason must have suffered a setback." When your baby moves into his incubator, remember that this is a good sign and another step forward.

Will My Baby Be Okay?

Within the first minute after every live premature birth, parents most naturally want to know, "Will my baby be okay?" "Will he have any physical or mental handicaps?" Unfortunately, it often requires at least two or three days of examinations and evaluation before the doctors can even begin to answer these questions realistically. But on that first day, once your baby has been thoroughly examined, once he has been hooked up to the monitors and his respiration is stabilized, his doctors will be able to talk with you about the state of his health at that moment. From there, one day at a time, you can keep track of his progress and hope for the best, knowing that preemies today have a tremendous advantage over those born just fifteen to twenty years ago. At that time, when a preemie was born, he was placed on a warming bed. Then, if he lived—he lived. If he died—he died. Today, immediate intensive care and high-quality research, along with major advances in medical technology, give doctors the knowledge and the tools they need to give preemies more than just a fighting chance. In hundreds of thousands of cases each year, we give them life.

SPECIAL PLACES

Where Are You Taking My Baby?

Over the past decade, hospital nurseries have been classified according to the level of care they can give to a newborn. The vast majority of hospitals in America are classified as Level I. The doctors at these hospitals can easily handle routine, uncomplicated labors and deliveries, and full-term healthy newborns. They are also equipped to deal with mild birth complications such as jaundice (see page 105), and can usually care for moderately premature babies over 35 weeks gestation and weighing at least 4 to 5 pounds. After the initial examination at a Level I hospital, a preemie's doctors may feel that he needs more intensive care than they are equipped to offer. In that case, he will be transported to a Level II or III hospital, which has the kind of equipment, technology, and personnel the baby needs.

A Level II hospital has the personnel and facilities to care for all but the smallest and sickest of premature babies. The extent to which the Level II facility will be prepared to do this varies depending upon many factors, including the demographics of the surrounding communities, its geographical location, the demand for intensive neonatal services, the referral patterns of the area hospitals, and its staff. Some Level II hospitals have a full-time neonatologist on staff. (This is a pediatrician who specializes in the care of newborns. See page 55 for a full discussion of this specialist.) This doctor can diagnose and treat many of the neonatal complications of premature birth. Although the exact cutoff age depends on the doctors' and the hospital's specific capabilities, the Level II hospital can usually manage mild to moderate cases of respiratory distress syndrome, and often has a special nursery equipped to care specifically for the needs of premature babies.

There are only 420 Level III hospitals in America at this

time. These hospitals are usually found in large cities and are often affiliated with large universities. They have fully equipped intensive care nurseries (ICNs), and are staffed with full-time neonatologists, as well as other specialists such as pediatric neurologists, surgeons, and developmentalists. These Level III hospitals are designated care centers for high-risk pregnancies, labors, and deliveries, and for newborns with severe medical and/or surgical problems.

The chart below will give you a quick comparative look at the three levels of hospital nurseries.

Hospital Nursery Levels

	Level I	*Level II*	*Level III*
Function	Risk assessment Management of uncomplicated perinatal care Stabilization of unexpected problems Initiation of maternal and neonatal transports	Level I plus: Diagnosis and treatment of some high-risk pregnancies and neonatal problems Initiation and acceptance of maternal-fetal and neonatal transports	Levels I and II plus: Diagnosis and treatment of all perinatal problems Acceptance of maternal-fetal and neonatal transports
Patients	Uncomplicated, emergency, and remedial problems such as lack of progress, immediate resuscitation of newborns, nursery care of large premature babies (over 4½ lbs., or 2000 q) without risk factors	Level I plus: Selected problems such as premature labor at 32 weeks and later, mild to moderate RDS, hypoglycemia, babies of diabetic mothers	Levels I and II plus: Premature rupture of membranes at 24 to 26 weeks, severe medical complications, prematurity at 32 to 36 weeks, severe RDS, babies with special needs such as prolonged mechanical ventilation

Chief of Service	One physician responsible for perinatal care (or codirectors from obstetrics and pediatrics)	Joint planning: Ob: Board-certified obstetrician with certification, special interest, experience, or training in maternal-fetal medicine Peds: Board-certified pediatrician with certification, special interest, experience, or training in neonatology	Codirectors: Ob: Full-time board-certified obstetrician with special competence in maternal-fetal medicine Peds: Full-time board-certified pediatrician with special competence in neonatal medicine
Other Physicians	Physician (or certified nurse-midwife) at all deliveries Anesthesia services Physician care for newborns	Level I plus: Board-certified director of anesthesia services Medical, surgical, radiology, pathology consultation	Levels I and II plus: Anesthesiologists with special training or experience in perinatal and pediatric anesthesia Obstetric and pediatric subspecialists
Supervisory Nurse	RN in charge of perinatal facilities	Ob: RN with education and experience in normal and high-risk pregnancy	Supervisor of perinatal services with advanced skills
		Peds: RN with education and experience in treatment of sick newborns	Separate head nurses for fetal and neonatal services

Hospital Nursery Levels *(continued)*

	Level I	*Level II*	*Level III*
Other Personnel	LPN, assistants under direction of head nurse	Level I plus: Social service, biomedical, respiratory therapy, laboratory as needed	Levels I and II plus: Designated and often full-time social service, respiratory therapy, biomedical engineering, laboratory technician, nurse-clinician, and specialists

Source: Adapted from *Guidelines for Perinatal Care* (Second Edition), American Academy of Pediatrics (Elk Grove Village, Ill.) and American College of Obstetricians and Gynecologists, (Washington, D.C.). Copyright 1988. Reprinted with permission.

Ideally, if a woman knows in advance that she is at risk for delivering prematurely (risk factors for premature delivery are discussed in Chapter Two), she will arrange for her baby to be born in a Level II or III hospital. Sometimes this means finding a new obstetrician and going far out of her way to an unfamiliar hospital, but the advantage that immediate and appropriate medical care can give to a preemie and to the mother makes the inconvenience well worthwhile.

If you're reading this book in advance of your delivery, there are a few things you should do to ensure the best care for your baby and yourself. Find out: (1) if your obstetrician has any reason to believe you may deliver prematurely, (2) the nursery level at the hospital where you plan to deliver, and (3) where the nearest Level II or III hospital is located. If your obstetrician can't refer you to a higher-level facility, you can get referral information by calling your State Health Society (Division of Maternal/Child Health). For national information on perinatal centers, you can call or write the National Perinatal Information Center in Providence, Rhode Island (1–401–274–0650). Also, if you are at risk for a premature birth, your obstetrician may refer you to a perinatologist. This is a doctor who has special training in the complications of pregnancy, labor, and delivery. He or she can monitor the problems of your pregnancy while you continue your routine visits to your own obstetrician.

If a preemie must be transported to another hospital, the transfer will be done in a methodical, prescribed manner that gives optimal attention to the baby's health and safety. After birth, at the hospital of delivery, the doctors will examine the baby, diagnose any problems, and take steps to correct complicating conditions to whatever extent they are able. They will also work to stabilize the preemie's body temperature, blood gas levels, blood pressure, and oxygen and blood sugar levels. These are important preparation procedures because a well-stabilized baby will require little or no treatment during transport.

The attending physician will explain to you the reasons for the baby's transfer and will ask for your written consent. You should also be given detailed information about the receiving hospital, such as the names of the staff members, the telephone number, and the visiting hours. If the hospital is a great distance away, you may even be given the names and location of places in the area where you can stay overnight.

Whether your baby is transported by ambulance, airplane, or helicopter, the vehicle will be specially equipped to act as a mini intensive care nursery. These transports always carry intensive care equipment, such as: transport incubator, oxygen supply, compressed air, oxygen hood, ventilation bag and mask, heart rate monitors, blood pressure unit, emergency drugs, and intravenous setup and solutions. A doctor, a nurse, and/or paramedics will make the trip with the baby to observe and monitor continually his body temperature, respiration and heart rate, blood pressure, color, activity, and oxygen concentrations.

The perinatal staff at the receiving hospital will be notified that your baby is on the way. A doctor and a nurse will meet the emergency vehicle the moment it arrives. Then the baby (still in his temperature-controlled, monitored, and stabilizing environment) will be taken to the hospital's ICN.

In this nursery, the preemie is examined again. His condition is reevaluated in consultation with the doctors from the hospital where he was born. Now, a specific plan of treatment will be formulated, and you will be filled in on the details.

Sometimes the baby's father will make the trip to the new hospital at the time of transport. There, he will be given up-to-date information on the diagnosis, treatment, and prognosis for the child. Most mothers (unless they, too, need critical intensive care) stay behind at the hospital of delivery to continue their own medical care and recuperation. In any event, whatever the physical arrangements, the mother is kept informed about her baby's state of health via the telephone, the baby's pediatrician (who has ongoing phone contact with the receiving physicians), and/or her spouse, who most often has the opportunity to be with the baby and talk directly to his doctors.

Sometimes, a preemie's doctors will arrange for his transfer several days, or even weeks, after his birth. This will happen when a preemie initially appears big enough and strong enough to stay in the Level I or II hospital where he is born, but later develops a complication that requires specialized treatment in a Level III ICN. Two days after Jason's birth, for example, just when Peggy and Bob were about ready to breathe the sigh of relief they had been holding back, the doctors noticed that Jason was experiencing frequent episodes of apnea, he was having digestive difficulties, and there was evidence of a brain hemorrhage. They decided to send him to an ICN at a Level III hospital forty miles away.

Peggy wasn't strong enough to go with Jason when he was first transferred because she was recovering from a cesarean delivery. "A doctor and a nurse brought Jason's portable incubator to the doorway of my hospital room, but they couldn't maneuver it over to my bed. They were in a hurry and I couldn't shuffle over there fast enough, so I blew Jason a hurried kiss good-bye, and then I sat back on my bed and cried for the next two hours. I remember I had this awful feeling that I wouldn't see Jason again. He looked so little and fragile, I couldn't imagine how he could pull through.

"On the first day, I didn't call the hospital at all because I didn't want to get bad news over the phone from a stranger. I wanted to wait for Bob to come back and tell me how Jason was doing, but it was so hard to wait. Every time I'd calm myself down and force myself to begin thinking positively, it would be time for the girl who was sharing the room with me to feed her baby and I'd start crying again. Seeing her baby was such a painful reminder of how sick my own baby was."

Jason's transfer to the ICN was difficult for Bob, too. "Peggy chose her obstetrician based on recommendation, location, and affiliation with a local hospital. We didn't know anything about the different levels of available care facilities; and we never thought to investigate them since we had no reason to believe anything would go wrong. All of a sudden, I had a critically ill son one hour's drive away, and a wife in another hospital who also needed me.

"Maybe this doesn't make a lot of sense, but I reacted by being angry. I was angry at Peggy for not knowing about this stuff in advance; I was angry at our doctors for not being able to take care of Jason; and I was angry at the doctors in the ICN because they seemed like intrusive strangers. Now I know the move was for the best and no one was to blame. But at the time it was hard to understand why it had to be that way. I thought a hospital was a hospital.

"When I first went to see Jason in the ICN, I was overwhelmed by the whole setup. There were about thirty-five preemies in incubators lined up in rows—all hooked up to monitors. The lights seemed so bright, the alarms so loud, and the people so hurried and businesslike. There was my son lying in the middle of all this, looking weak and frail. I stood next to his incubator and stared at him for about a half hour. I tried to memorize every inch of his being— every facial feature, each little finger, his tiny feet, and every strand of his beautiful black hair. I wanted to be sure that if he died that day, I'd always have a clear picture of my son in my mind. When it was time for me to leave, I had this nagging feeling that Jason would be lonely in that crowded room. When I was out in the parking lot, I got an idea. I doubled back to the hospital's giftshop, bought a teddy bear, brought it back to the nursery, and put it in his incubator. It somehow made me feel better knowing he had company."

How long a preemie will stay in the ICN depends on his individual needs. Some babies stay in the Level II or III intensive care nursery for only a few days; others stay for weeks, and some stay for months. Eventually, when their condition is no longer critical, when they no longer need the highly specialized equipment and care found in the ICN, they are usually sent back to the hospital where they were born. Here, in a place where their vital signs are stabilized and monitored, they are given the extra time they need to grow strong enough to go home.

In the future, more hospitals will be able to upgrade their nurseries to be classified as Level II or III facilities. This will reduce the number of preemies who must be transported to hospitals far from home. But for now, if your baby is transported to an intensive care nursery in another hospital, (although it's quite natural for you to feel anxious about the move) you should remember that it is an opportunity for him to receive the very best care today's medical community can offer.

SPECIAL PEOPLE

When a child is born prematurely there are usually four people who are routinely and immediately involved in his care. These professionals make up what is called the primary-care team. Then, if extraordinary complications develop, there are other medical specialists who may be called in to work with the baby. These professionals comprise the secondary-care team. Although each member of the primary and secondary teams has a specific and specialized job to do, their responsibilities interweave in an intricate pattern of neonatal care that gives thorough and comprehensive medical attention to a preemie.

Primary-Care Team

Neonatologist

The neonatologist is a physician who specializes in the development, care, and diseases of newborns. This medical doctor also has special training and expertise in the complications of pregnancy, labor, and delivery (such as premature labor and birth) that may negatively affect a baby. The neonatologist will routinely care for all premature babies born weighing less than 3 to 4 pounds, and also for heavier babies who have breathing difficulties and/or severe health complications.

Neonatology is a relatively new field of medicine; it was first officially recognized by the American Academy of Pediatrics in 1975. The emergence of this subspeciality over the past fifteen years, along with improved equipment and care procedures, is the reason why today's preemie survival rates are far superior to those of years ago. (A recent study has found that in 1960 the survival rate for preemies born weighing less than 3 pounds 5 ounces was 27 percent. Today it is 72 percent.*) However, because neonatology is a highly specialized field of medicine, not all hospitals have the staff or the equipment to support a comprehensive neonatal program. That is why, as explained earlier, preemies born in a hospital without an in-house neonatologist may be transported to a Level II or III facility.

At these hospitals a neonatologist will take primary responsibility for the care of a preemie. He or she is generally present during a preterm delivery, and after birth he or she will resuscitate the infant (if necessary), and stabilize the body temperature and breathing and heart rates. On a daily basis, the neonatologist will examine, evaluate, and treat problems associated with prematurity such as apnea, bradycardia, and/or respiratory difficulties. He or she will arrange for the appropriate feeding method, and will decide if and when IV fluids should be given. This doctor will also decide what treatment procedures are most appropriate, arrange for round-the-clock observa-

---

*U.S. Congress, Office of Technology Assessment, *Health Technology Case Study 38: Neonatal Intensive Care for Low Birthweight Babies—Costs and Effectiveness* (Washington, D.C.: United States Government Printing Office, December 1987).

tion, and then initiate and coordinate the efforts of all other medical personnel who will be involved in caring for the infant.

The neonatologist knows that it is difficult for you to relinquish control of your baby's care to a doctor who, in most cases, is completely unknown to you. When he or she initially takes over the care of your baby, the neonatologist will acknowledge your need for assurance and information by carefully explaining to you the details of your baby's condition. He or she will describe all treatments, tests, and evaluative procedures, and answer all your questions. He or she will explain why your baby is attached to monitor wires and when they will be removed. The neonatologist will also explain anticipated problems and the sequence of events you can expect in the first few days or weeks. However, after this introductory meeting, the neonatologist's long-term involvement with you and your family will depend on the particular doctor, hospital, and on the baby's condition.

In Level III teaching hospitals (those affiliated with universities), a neonatologist will be a preemie's primary attending physician. He or she will be in the nursery for approximately one hour, five to seven days a week, making rounds to examine every preemie under his or her care. The neonatologist will make these rounds with the fellows, interns, and residents (see Glossary) who are assigned to the nursery at that time. Together they will discuss babies who have special problems, and those new to the nursery. During the rest of the day the neonatologists are assigned to teaching and research duties. This kind of schedule may make it difficult for the neonatologist to be available for informal parent conferences. If a baby has special problems and is in need of extraordinary care, the neonatologist will certainly meet with the family to explain these problems, but generally your day-to-day parent/doctor discussions will be with the fellows, residents, and interns.

If it should happen that you can't get answers to your questions because of the neonatologists' hectic schedules, or because the fellows, residents, and/or interns do not seem to be completely up-to-date on your baby's condition—don't despair. The other members of the primary-care team described below should certainly be able to keep you fully informed. Also, if you have a particular concern that you want to discuss with the neonatologist, don't hesitate to call his or her office and make an appointment. Even though busy schedules may limit their ability to address personally all of your questions on a daily basis, neonatologists give your baby the very best care possible, and if you ask, they will make time to meet and talk with you.

In smaller, nonteaching hospitals, neonatologists usually have a schedule that allows them a closer and more personal relationship with the baby's entire family. Because these doctors do not have to do as many teaching rounds, you may be able to meet them in the nursery each day when it's time for your baby's examination. If you have the opportunity to do this, watch how the neonatologist handles the baby (this will assure you that preemies don't break if you pick them up); ask questions about the baby's condition (bring a written list so you won't forget to mention what's on your mind); and ask the neonatologist to show you how you can become more involved in the care of your baby. It takes time to learn all about premature baby care and to adjust to your new role as the parent of a preemie. In nonteaching hospitals, the neonatologist is more readily available to help you do both of these things.

If your baby is in a nonteaching hospital, take advantage of the accessibility of the neonatologist. If you can't be in the nursery when he or she is there, ask if you can arrange for a daily phone conference. Once you get over the initial panic of expecting the worst when you hear the neonatologist's voice on the phone, a routine two-minute report will help to calm your nerves and keep you from dwelling on the horrible "what-ifs" that may creep into your mind when you haven't heard any news for a while. If you have a major concern that you want to discuss personally, ask for an appointment. It's usually better if you arrange to meet in a place outside the nursery, where the neonatologist isn't subject to continuous interruptions and distractions.

Whether your baby is being cared for in a large university hospital or in a smaller non-teaching hospital, the neonatologists will give your baby the same kind of intensive, high-quality care. They will do this in conjunction with the other members of the primary-care team described below. If there is reason to suspect that your baby needs some form of intensive medical intervention, the appropriate pediatric specialist will be asked to evaluate the child and confer with the neonatologist on a plan of action. (A description of some secondary-care specialists appears later in this chapter.) When this is the case, the neonatologist will again be the one to explain to you the baby's condition, and the reason for bringing in a specialist. The neonatologist will be able to answer all your questions about the proposed procedure, but if you would like, he or she can also arrange for you to talk directly to the specialist.

The neonatologist will remain responsible for your baby's care for as long as is required. This is usually until the child is completely stable and his care is transferred to the pediatrician, until he is stable enough to be sent back to the hospital of his birth, or until he is discharged from the hospital and (finally!) sent home to you.

Pediatrician

A pediatrician is a physician who specializes in the development, care, and diseases of children. Although the pediatrician's work with the complications of premature birth is less specialized than that of the neonatologist, this doctor has a good and solid understanding of newborn care (both full-term and premature), and is very much a part of your baby's primary-care team.

The immediate role of the pediatrician in the care of a premature infant depends on the baby's gestational age, birth weight, and place of birth. If a woman goes into labor at or after 35 weeks gestation, and it appears that the baby will weigh at least 5 pounds, the pediatrician will usually be responsible for the baby's care regardless of whether he is born in a Level I, II, or III hospital.

If, however, a woman delivers before the thirty-fifth week, the role of the pediatrician depends on the level of the hospital in which the child is born, and if the baby is transported out to an intensive care nursery. In a Level I hospital (or a Level II that does not have an in-house neonatologist) the pediatrician is the doctor responsible for the baby's care at birth. He or she will examine and evaluate, diagnose and stabilize, prescribe treatment, and decide if the preemie needs to be transported to a Level II or III facility and which one will best serve the child's needs. (General practice dictates that any baby who needs breathing assistance, or who is born weighing less than 4 pounds, should be transferred to a higher-level facility so that, ideally, he will be in the ICN *before* major complications become evident.) If the baby does not need to be transported to another hospital, the pediatrician will take full responsibility for his care. If the preemie does need higher-level care, the pediatrician will stay with him until the transport team arrives.

The pediatrician will also spend time with the baby's parents. He or she will carefully explain the baby's condition, and if necessary, the reasons for transfer based on the limitations of the hospital facilities and of the pediatrician him- or herself (unlike hospitals with neonatologists on staff, the pediatrician cannot personally watch your baby's progress twenty-four hours a day). In most cases, after the baby is moved out, the pediatrician will continue to visit the mother every day while she remains in the hospital. Because the pediatrician maintains phone contact with the neonatologist at the receiving hospital, he or she will keep the mother informed and will explain the details of her baby's medical condition.

If the mother is discharged from the hospital while the baby is still in the ICN at another hospital, the pediatrician's active caretaking role diminishes for a while. Most neonatologists, however, will maintain contact with the sending pediatrician throughout the baby's stay. This ongoing communication is very important because the pediatrician will regain charge of the baby's health when he is sent home from the ICN, or when he returns to the hospital of birth for follow-up care.

If the neonatologists are not initiating this kind of discourse with your pediatrician—speak up. Some Level III facilities have excellent reputations for keeping close contact with the sending pediatrician; others, unfortunately, are known to be lax in this communication. Let the neonatologist know that you want your pediatrician kept up-to-date on the status of the baby's health. Then check with the pediatrician to be sure he or she knows what's going on. If the neonatologists don't report back to the pediatrician, you should ask the pediatrician to initiate the contact. A well-informed pediatrician will also enhance your own understanding of your baby's condition. Because pediatricians follow the graduates of ICNs through to their teen years, they can sometimes give invaluable insight into some generally expected outcomes of birth complications. If he or she is kept informed, you will have another medical expert to turn to for information, explanations, and even comfort.

When a preemie is born at the same Level III hospital (or a Level II with an in-house neonatologist) where the family's pediatrician is also on staff, the parents sometimes become confused about who's taking care of the baby. Very often they ask, "If the neonatologist is now my baby's doctor, what does the pediatrician do?" Or, "Which doctor, the neonatologist or the pediatrician, should I call when I have a question?" Or, "Since there is a specialist caring for my baby in the hospital, should I wait until the baby goes home to choose a pediatrician?"

Although it may initially be a bit confusing, the ideal situation is where a premature baby is born in a hospital where both a neonatologist and the family's chosen pediatrician are practicing. In this case, the doctors can work together to give the preemie the advantage of dual coverage. The neonatologist has the ultimate responsibility for the baby's care as long as he needs respiratory assistance and/or is still experiencing any complications of the premature birth (e.g., inability to self-regulate body temperature, breathing pauses, or irregular heartbeat patterns). Even during this time, however, the neonatologist will work closely with the pediatrician, and they will continually confer on diagnosis and treatment procedures. Since both the neonatologist and the pediatrician will be monitoring your baby's health every day, either one (or both!) can answer your questions.

On the other hand, the role of the pediatrician in caring for a preemie is initially very limited when the infant is born in a hospital other than the one where he or she practices. When this is the case, the parents should tell the attending doctors to contact their pediatrician to alert him or her to the premature birth. They should also insist that the pediatrician be kept informed throughout the course of the baby's hospital stay. Then, when the baby is discharged from the hospital of birth, the pediatrician will be ready to pick up his care right where the neonatologist left off.

When your preemie is discharged from the hospital, the pediatrician will take full charge of his health. He or she will keep close watch on the child's progress and growth by scheduling checkups at regular intervals. All secondary specialists (listed below) who may still be involved in caring for your baby will confer with and report back to the pediatrician. Also, any at-home nursing care, respirators, or monitors will be dispensed through the pediatrician.

The pediatrician is usually the only member of the primary-care team whom you can handpick. Since this person will monitor your baby's growth and development for many years, he or she should certainly be a person whom you trust without reservation and with whom you can develop a good rapport. Actually, it's a good idea to begin this search in the very beginning of a pregnancy, especially if you know you are at risk for delivering prematurely. (If you deliver before you have chosen a pediatrician, one of the hospital's pediatric staff members will be assigned to your baby. Then, as soon as possible, make sure you choose the one you personally want to care for your baby.) It is also a good idea to choose a pediatrician early in your pregnancy because he or she may be helpful in locating an appropriate ICN, and may be able to recommend an obstetrician skilled in handling high-risk pregnancies.

When you look for a pediatrician you will find that, today, most are members of group practices, which means there is more than one physician to consider when making your decision. It is a mistake to choose a group if you love one of the doctors but abhor the others. That one doctor will not always be available to you, will not do rounds in the hospital every day, and may not be the one on duty when a crisis arises. Look for a group that has a uniform approach to pediatric care; a group that follows the same procedures for the same ailments; a group that insists on good communication among its members by passing all case documents around for review by each doctor; a group that won't treat you like a small part of a big business; a group who has formulated a philosophy of teamwork that will meet your needs no matter who is in the office when you have an appointment.

If you don't like the idea of taking your baby to a pediatric group, call the head of pediatrics at your local hospital and ask for a referral to a pediatrician who is in solo practice. These pediatricians are still around. Keep looking until you find the person who fits your needs.

Choose your pediatrician carefully, thoughtfully, and early. This is the one member of the primary-care team who is in it for the long haul—right through to the teen years.

Primary-Care Nurses

The primary-care neonatal nurses are responsible for the minute-to-minute, individualized care of your baby. These nurses have training in and experience with the special needs of premature babies (as well as full-term babies with medical complications). They are the round-the-clock eyes and ears of the doctors, and they do 80 to 90 percent of the ongoing work with the baby's family.

When your baby's primary nurse comes on duty, she will first read over his chart. (Because most primary-care nurses are female, we will use the feminine pronoun in this section.) This will alert her to any specific problems (such as apnea episodes, digestive difficulties, excessive crying) that may require attentive follow-up care and/or close monitoring. Then the nurse will begin her routine procedures, observations, and evaluations, which will then be carefully documented on the baby's chart and repeated periodically as ordered by the neonatologist or pediatrician.

This routine care involves thorough checking of the sensors and monitors that give heart, respiratory, and body temperature information. It also includes personal observation of the baby's skin tone, behavior, IV insertion sites, and any changes in the baby's physical condition. The nurse will provide, measure, and record the baby's food intake (whether given through IV, NG tube, or nipple). She will also measure and record the output of urine and feces. It is the nurse's job as well to monitor lab work, gather the results, and report them to the physician. And each day, during one of the shifts, a nurse will bathe and weigh the baby.

Neonatal nurses are also trained to perform many medical procedures that are sometimes necessary in the day-to-day care of your baby. They may need to do a chest percussion, for example, to loosen secretions and make sure the lungs are well aerated. Also, if a preemie needs to be moved to another part of the hospital (for surgery, X-rays, and such) a nurse will accompany the baby so she can continually monitor his vital signs. When necessary, she can administer medication, insert IV lines, and draw blood samples from the baby's heel. (In some hospitals, the nurse also may be permitted to draw the blood back from an umbilical artery line.) All nursery nurses are trained to administer CPR and use a resuscitation bag to stimulate or resuscitate babies experiencing breathing difficulties. If your baby shows signs of distress, the primary nurse is the person who is on the spot to stabilize him and call for the physician's help when needed.

In addition to this kind of hands-on physical care, the primary nurse plays a vital role in teaching you how to parent your baby comfortably and confidently. She knows that when you first enter the nursery, you may feel out of place. It can be awkward to visit your baby in a strange environment where everyone except you seems to know what he or she is doing. When you feel this way, remember that, although all these professional people efficiently care for your baby's physical health, only you can give him the kind of time, attention, and love he needs to grow. Because the nurse spends more time with your baby than anyone else in the hospital, she is the best person to tell you all about your baby's need for attention, his moods, his appetite, his sleep patterns, and even his personality. She will show you how, and then encourage you, to handle, touch, massage, talk, feed, and love your baby even when he can't yet leave his incubator. (See Chapter Eight for a detailed explanation of how to do these things.)

The nurses know that your baby needs you and that you need to be with your baby. When you visit the nursery, you are not intruding on their territory or interrupting their work. In fact, the nurses will be glad to tell you when your baby will be awake, and when he will be bathed, changed, weighed, and fed each day so you can arrange to visit at these times and stay actively involved in his care. Helping you feel comfortable in the nursery and with your baby is an important part of their job. You are not in the way— you are a part of the whole picture.

The primary nurse is also a valuable source of information. Although the doctors can best explain the scientific basis for your baby's treatment and care, the nurses can give you an up-to-the-minute progress report anytime you want one. If you wake in the middle of the night in need of reassurance, you can call the nursery and ask to speak to the nurse who is handling your baby. You'll get an honest and complete report without any need to apologize for calling; just as you are concerned about your baby twenty-four hours a day, the nurses are there twenty-four hours a day to give him medical care. They know that because they are the most accessible primary-care team members, they are the ones you will turn to most often for information, guidance, and comfort.

The primary nurses are also the ones who are there with the baby when you can't be. At these times, it would not be unusual for the nurse to try to supplement your baby's need for attention by gently stroking him, talking to him, and when possible, rocking him and holding him close to kiss his brow. These nurses are the closest person to you whom your baby will know during this time away from home. That's probably why, when a preemie is discharged, you'll see many nurses struggling to hold back their tears as they send a little bit of themselves home with the baby.

Social Worker

The primary function of a social worker in an intensive care nursery is to give supportive counseling and emotional encouragement to you, the baby's parents. In all Level III and some Level II nurseries, a social worker will contact you (usually within twenty-four hours of the baby's birth) to assess your needs and try to help you deal with any medical, personal, family, or financial problems. For example:

1. A social worker will talk with you to determine if you have complete and correct information about the state of your baby's health, and about your role in his care. He or she will act as a go-between for you and the baby's doctors and nurses. This social worker will help you to understand better and accept what the doctors tell you, and he or she will also encourage you to become an active member of your baby's primary-care team.

2. If you are not pleased with the way the doctors and nurses are caring for your baby, the social worker will listen to your concerns and convey them to the professionals involved. He or she may arrange a meeting outside the nursery for you and the appropriate doctor and/or nurse. Sometimes, just being away from the nursery environment and talking out your concerns will help put things in their proper perspective. The social worker will then continue to talk to the doctors for you until the problem issues are resolved.

3. A social worker is trained to assess how well you and/ or your spouse are coping with the premature birth and consequent problems. If you are having difficulties, he or

she will encourage you to talk about your fears and concerns, and then will teach you coping skills to help you better deal with the situation.

4. A social worker can ease the way for parents who are hesitant about seeing, touching, or holding their baby. He or she will go into the nursery with the parents to lend support, encouragement, and know-how. If a parent still feels unsure about seeing the baby, the social worker may take a picture of the baby to allow the parent a private preview before meeting the baby in the nursery.

5. Parents of preemies need a strong support system of family and friends to help them through the difficult days. At first, however, family and friends may withhold their support because they don't know whether to offer congratulations or condolences. The ICN social workers understand that this often happens and will be there to listen to and talk with you. They will not attempt to minimize your feelings; they will assure you that what you are going through is normal. Because they have a clear understanding of your baby's medical situation, they can also help keep you in touch with reality.

6. Social workers also offer their counseling services to the preemie's brothers and sisters and grandparents. The social worker will help these relatives understand what is happening to the new baby, and will work with any family member who is afraid to visit the hospital, or who is scared by the nursery environment.

7. If you are in need of social or financial assistance, the social worker will give you information about programs such as the Women, Infants, and Children program (WIC), which supplies vouchers for food items, the family-focused Bureau of Child Welfare or the Division of Youth and Family Services, the State Department Board of Health, local parent support groups, Medicaid, and Supplemental Security Income. He or she can also help you decipher your

own insurance policy, contact your insurance agent, and evaluate the coverage you currently have.

8. The social worker is very involved at the time of your baby's discharge. He or she will assess your readiness to continue your baby's care at home. If appropriate, the social worker will arrange for visiting nurse services, early intervention program visits, and a follow-up support system. He or she may also be instrumental in easing the transition from neonatal care to pediatric care.

Social workers wear many hats, but in all their jobs, they are an unfaltering source of encouragement and support (something parents of preemies can always use!). If you are not contacted by a social worker, tell your doctor you would like to meet with someone from the social services department. This is the member of the primary-care team who cares for YOU, the parents of the preemie.

Secondary-Care Team

Audiologist

An audiologist is a medical professional who is specially trained to detect, diagnose, and treat individuals with impaired hearing. Ideally, an audiologist will examine the hearing capabilities of all premature babies at some point in their first year, but most commonly, he or she is called in by the child's attending physician only when there is reason to suspect hearing loss.

It is very difficult to detect hearing loss in a newborn through clinical observations. However, there are a number of prematurity-related conditions that are known to affect the infant's hearing sometimes and that, when present, will warrant an auditory examination. These conditions include intraventricular hemorrhage (page 99), bacterial meningitis (page 97), severe jaundice (page 106), cranial or facial disorders, prolonged use of certain ototoxic antibiotics, and/ or a family history of hearing impairment.

The audiological examination performed in the nursery is called evoked potential testing (also called auditory brain stem response studies, or brain stem auditory evoked response studies). This is an electrodiagnostic procedure in which electrodes are attached to the skin on the baby's head in a noninvasive manner with a conductive paste. Clicking sounds are presented through earphones to the baby's ears. The sounds are used to evoke a response pattern between the auditory nerve and the midbrain. This response is observed and measured, and gives audiologists the information they need to determine the baby's potential for hearing high-frequency sounds. If this testing procedure indicates any level of hearing impairment, the child will be tested again in three months (or possibly sooner if there are changes in the baby's medical status) to see if there is a change in the potential as the baby's brain stem and cardiopulmonary systems mature. If the hearing problem is still evident (as is the case in approximately 2 to 4 percent of preemies), the audiologist may initiate intervention for rehabilitation. This may include a hearing aid evaluation, referral to medical specialists, and/or placement in an early intervention program that is sensitive to the needs of the hearing impaired.

In many states, regardless of the outcome of the initial auditory evaluation, children who experience any of the above-mentioned conditions associated with hearing loss are automatically referred to a state auditory screening registry. Through this registry, the child's parents are advised to schedule frequent hearing checkups. Even when the auditory exam performed in the nursery finds no evidence of hearing impairment, the child's hearing should be checked again (ideally at about the age of six months) with behavioral tests that record responses to specific frequencies in sound. Some children may appear to have full auditory functioning, but, in fact, may have a low-frequency hearing loss or a high-frequency hearing loss that would allow them to appear to respond appropriately to environmental sounds but might significantly impair their speech and language development.

If the neonatologist feels it is necessary for your baby to have an auditory examination, ask for an appointment (or at least a phone conference) with the audiologist to discuss future hearing evaluations. Too often detection of subtle hearing impairment is delayed until the child is older and his speech pattern indicates a problem. Early detection of hearing loss and corrective intervention in infancy are now available for your baby; if necessary, take advantage of the opportunity.

Pediatric Neurologist

A neurologist is a pediatrician skilled and trained in the diagnosis and treatment of diseases of the nervous system as they pertain to infants and children. As medical technology advances, the vital question in the event of a premature birth is often no longer, "Will my baby survive?," but rather, "Will he be normal?" The neurologist is the person who can help the neonatologist answer that question for you.

It is difficult to say in what capacity the neurologist will be involved in the care of your child because ICNs can set their own policies in this regard. Some routinely have all preemies examined by a neurologist; others may call for a neurological examination only if there is reason to suspect a problem. Either way, the neonatologist will remain alert to any signs of neurological damage and will consult with the neurologist any time he or she suspects a problem.

Indications of such problems may include: seizures, severe respiratory distress syndrome, severe or extended apnea, paralysis on one side of the body, genetic disorders (such as Down's Syndrome), brain hemorrhage, abnormal

increase in the amount of fluid within the brain cavity (hydrocephalus), deficient muscle tone (hypotonia), abnormal
movements such as persistent shaking, unusual feeding or
sleeping problems, or metabolic problems such as high
sugar and/or ammonia levels, or low sugar and/or calcium
levels. (See "Complications" on page 82 for a full discussion of some of these problems.)

When a neurologist comes to examine your baby, he or
she will test observable signs such as motor strength, body
and extremity movement, reflex movements, degree of
muscle tone and flexibility, the ability to coordinate sucking and swallowing, and the degree to which the baby can
look at a person and follow his or her face as it moves
away. The neurologist will also examine a preemie when
he is full-term corrected age. At that time he or she will
assess the baby's tone, posture, and reflexes. He will note
if the baby has difficulty moving his body, or is arching
his back abnormally, or has trouble holding his head up,
or has an abnormal cry. All of these things will help the
neurologist evaluate the baby's maturity and assess the consequences of his medical problems.

It is usually very difficult to determine with absolute certainty to what degree neurological problems in the infant
preemie will have long-term effects. Because so much of
the premature brain is still developing, it is sometimes a
slow wait-and-see kind of prognosis. Some neurological de-
ficiencies and abnormalities in a preemie will correct themselves as the child grows and matures. Others can be
rectified or compensated for with neurosurgery or with the
help of physical therapy. (When these recourses are necessary, the neurologist will make the appropriate arrangements.) And still other neurological problems may
permanently affect the child's mental and/or physical functioning. In the 1960s about 70 percent of high-risk premature infants had significant handicapping problems. Today,

only 5 to 15 percent of babies weighing between 2 pounds 4 ounces and 3 pounds 5 ounces will have these problems (which include cerebral palsy and cognitive delays). About 30 percent of babies weighing less than 1 pound 12 ounces show these signs of significant developmental problems, while between 20 and 30 percent will grow to have mild developmental problems such as speech and language difficulties, coordination problems, behavior problems (especially attention deficit disorder), and learning difficulties.

It is certainly understandable why the parents of premature babies are anxious for a definitive answer to the question, "Will my baby be normal?," but in the domain of neurological development one must try especially hard to accept the state of the baby's physical and mental health as it matures one day at a time.

Developmental Pediatrician

A developmental pediatrician is a specially trained medical doctor who is primarily concerned with the evaluation of children who are at risk and who may show signs of developmental problems. These kinds of problems might include a lag in motor coordination skills (such as lifting the head up, rolling over, sitting, standing, and walking), hearing or vision impairment, behavioral problems such as extreme irritability or inconsolability, and learning disabilities.

It is the developmental pediatrician who will determine if your baby's developmental progress is on par with his corrected-age expectations. For example, if a baby is born eight weeks before his due date, it is perfectly normal for his developmental skills to fall two months behind where they would have been if he were born at term. This baby may not be able to roll over when he is four months old (like his older full-term brother did), but the developmentalist would expect he could do this at six months of age, which is an appropriate schedule for his four-months corrected age.

Some severe developmental problems such as retardation or cerebral palsy may be evident within the first few weeks or months of life (especially with preemies who weigh less than 3½ pounds). When the neonatologist or pediatrician notices that a baby is persistently irritable, or stiff, or too easily startled, or shows no interest in the human face, or shows lack of response to sound, he or she may contact the developmentalist as well as the neurologist to examine the baby. If at this time the developmentalist can see a developmental delay, he or she may schedule periodic reevaluations to monitor progress or deterioration. The developmentalist may ask a physical therapist or the primary nurse to provide the baby with opportunities for visual and physical stimulation, which may encourage developmental growth. He or she may also encourage you to help stimulate the baby while he is still in his incubator with things like toys, mobiles, prescribed exercises, and soothing music.

The majority of preemies will not see a developmentalist while they are in the hospital. Because "normalcy" is generally judged according to the baby's corrected age and in comparison to what he should be doing if he were born on his due date, most often the developmentalist will become involved in the baby's care when he is approximately three-months corrected age. At this time he or she will begin to evaluate your baby's physical and mental capabilities and will teach you how to help your child reach and maintain an optimal level of performance. Most developmentalists will schedule routine follow-up visits at least through the early school years, because mild or moderate developmental problems may not be evident for months or even years after birth.

Pediatric Cardiologist

Pediatric cardiologists are physicians who are specially trained in the diagnosis and treatment of heart conditions in children. These doctors have completed the general course of internship and residency in pediatric training, and a fellowship in pediatric cardiology. Their work is highly specialized and there are only approximately seven hundred pediatric cardiologists certified by the American Academy of Pediatrics today.

If a preemie's attending physicians suspect a cardiac problem, they will call in a pediatric cardiologist for a consultation. These suspected problems may include a persistent blue skin color without an apparent explanation, congestive heart failure whereby the heart is not pumping adequately, an irregular heart rhythm, or an infection that seems to be affecting the functioning of the heart. The cardiologist will examine the baby and confer with the neonatologist on a plan of diagnostic tests that may include X-rays, echocardiogram, EKG, cardiac catheterization, and blood gas determinations. If a cardiac problem is found, the cardiologist will determine appropriate treatment. If the baby needs heart surgery, a pediatric cardiovascular surgeon will join the medical care team.

Pediatric cardiologists are usually affiliated with higher-level medical centers. If a baby is born in a lower-level facility and the doctors there suspect a heart problem, the child will be transferred to the nearest Level II or III hospital that has a pediatric cardiologist on staff.

If a pediatric cardiologist is called in to examine a baby, he or she may not personally meet with the baby's parents. For lesser heart problems that require routine diagnosis and noninvasive treatment, the cardiologist will tend to the baby each day when making rounds, and the neonatologist will continue the ongoing communication with the parents.

However, if a baby has a true structural heart deformity that needs more intensive workup, care, or surgical intervention, or that may ultimately be a long-term problem, the cardiologist will certainly meet with the parents to explain the situation and map out a course of diagnosis, management, and long-term care. The pediatric cardiologist is one more member of the medical care team who will ensure that your baby has the very best, most up-to-date, and highly specialized care available.

Pediatric Ophthalmologist

An ophthalmologist is a medical doctor who can diagnose and treat injuries or defects that affect the eyes. He or she can prescribe glasses and medication and can perform surgery.

Before your baby is discharged, this doctor will examine his eyes to check for prematurity-related retinal problems. If your baby will be in the nursery for an extended period of time, his eyes will first be examined at five or six weeks of age. This examination is necessary because one third of all premature infants (especially those weighing less than 2 pounds 4 ounces at birth) develop an eye problem called retinopathy of prematurity (page 120). This condition involves the retina and the blood vessels that run over its surface to supply oxygen and nourishment.

You will probably be told when this exam is going to take place, but the ophthalmologist will generally pass his or her findings along to you through the neonatologist. If there is a problem, or if you have a particular concern, you can certainly arrange for a personal meeting. If upon discharge your baby's retina and/or blood vessels are still not completely matured, the ophthalmologist will schedule follow-up visits at his or her office.

Pediatric Radiologist

A pediatric radiologist is a medical doctor who has been specially trained to perform and interpret radiographic and ultrasonographic procedures as they are used to diagnose problems of infants and children. There are only four hundred to five hundred board-certified pediatric radiologists in the United States and Canada, so it is possible that one may not be on staff at your baby's hospital. In this case, it will be necessary for staff radiologists to be involved in the ongoing care and evaluation of your baby's health, which very often includes the use of procedures such as sonograms and X-rays.

Sonograms and X-rays are painless, noninvasive ways to evaluate a baby's condition; most often they can be performed right in the nursery so the baby doesn't have to be moved. Although you will probably never meet the radiologists who are involved in the care of your preemie, they are in continual contact with the neonatologist and are very much a part of the medical care team and you should know what they do.

Some diagnostic procedures are performed as routine precautionary measures. For example, a sonogram (also called an ultrasound) of the brain is usually performed on babies less than 34 weeks gestational age (or those weighing less than 4 pounds) to check for a brain hemorrhage. A sonogram may also be used if the neonatologist suspects problems in other parts of the body, such as the heart, muscles, joints, hip, kidneys, gastrointestinal tract, liver, gallbladder, or urinary tract. (Sonograms are usually the first means of examination because they are noninvasive and do not use radiation.)

A type of sonogram that may be used to examine your baby's heart is an echocardiogram. This procedure combines many related sonographic methods such as Doppler and color techniques. The complete echocardiogram lets the doctors look at the structure and function of the heart.

In full color, it gives them information about the direction of the blood flow and the amount of blood going to and from the heart. This ultrasonographic procedure often allows doctors to avoid the more complicated and dangerous surgical insertion of a cardiac catheter.

Because sonograms cannot show calcium or pockets of air in and around tissues and organs, X-rays will be taken when there is a need to examine a preemie's bones, lungs, and/or intestinal tract. They may also be taken to check on the position of any tubes or catheters inside the baby's body.

When X-rays are taken in the nursery, the doctors, nurses, and parents usually leave the room to avoid radiation exposure. This, of course, may make you wonder about the harmful effects the X-rays might have on the baby being examined as well as on those in neighboring incubators. The amount of radiation that enters the body with one X-ray is minimal; the radiation scatter that may touch surrounding babies is barely measurable or nonexistent. But most importantly, the radiation from X-rays does not stay in the body; after a day or less, all effects of radiation should be gone. The danger in exposure occurs when the radiation is repeatedly absorbed into the body over a long period of time without waiting for the effects to dissipate. That's why leaving the room may be appropriate for the nurses and doctors who would endure daily exposure over the years. Most likely, your baby could have one or possibly more X-rays every day over the course of a couple of weeks without experiencing any harmful effects. The X-ray technician may ask you to leave the room because it is common practice, or hospital policy, or even state law. But because of today's methods of delivering minimal amounts of radiation, you would probably not be in danger if you stayed (and should not be alarmed by the procedure).

There are other radiographic procedures that, although

not routinely performed on premature babies, may be used to evaluate specific complications. Some of these are discussed in Chapter Three.

It is the pediatric radiologist who will read and interpret the results of all these tests. When your baby is given one of these procedures, his doctors may tell you that they must speak to the radiologist before they can discuss the results. This is because the most accurate and comprehensive report is compiled by merging the radiologist's special training in reading and interpreting these tests with the neonatologist's knowledge of your child's specific health condition.

Respiratory Therapist

Respiratory therapists are specially trained to set up, calibrate, monitor, and supervise the use of the respiratory equipment in the nursery. For example, if your baby needs an oxygen hood, CPAP therapy, or a respirator (these pieces of respiratory equipment are explained on pages 33–36), it is the respiratory therapist who will set up the equipment, make sure it is functioning properly, and set the dials to the appropriate breathing rate, air pressure, oxygen, and humidity prescribed by the doctor. The respiratory therapist is also responsible for analyzing the air going through the tubes to make sure it equals the settings the doctor ordered. When necessary, he or she will also set up the pulse oximeter or other monitors and then place the sensors on the baby's body.

Once the respiratory therapist has confirmed that the equipment is working as it should and that the baby is getting exactly what has been prescribed, he or she will monitor the equipment approximately every two to four hours (or more if necessary) and will record the findings on the respiratory therapy chart attached to the machine. (This documentation helps the doctors make patterned correlations between the nurses' dated notes about the baby's general health and the source and amount of oxygen being administered at any given time.)

The respiratory therapist also plays a role in infection control by ensuring that all the respiratory equipment is cleaned appropriately and changed frequently to prevent bacterial contamination. As a general rule, all equipment will be changed by the respiratory therapist every twenty-four to forty-eight hours.

In a Level III (or a sophisticated Level II) hospital, a therapist is a permanent member of the intensive care nursery staff and is always in the ICN. This provides for immediate attention to any sudden respiratory problem, and it also allows for quick and proficient analysis of blood gases, which can be done by the therapist right in the nursery. The doctors in the higher care facilities need fast reaction to respiratory problems because they are caring for smaller, more critically ill infants than are in the Level I or II facility. In a Level I or Level II nursery, the respiratory therapy equipment is also well maintained, and blood gas analysis can also be done when necessary. The respiratory therapists in these hospitals will make rounds in the nurseries every few hours, but they usually do not stay there throughout the day, and so are not always immediately available. When blood gases are drawn, they must be put on ice and sent to the lab. The results are then called up to the nursery a few minutes later. This is another reason why babies who need intensive respiratory care should be in a Level II or III nursery.

Regardless of the hospital level, when a preemie needs respiratory assistance, the respiratory therapist becomes an invaluable member of the medical team.

Other Health Care Providers

The people who make up the primary- and secondary-care teams are those most actively involved in caring for your baby. There are other behind-the-scenes people, however, who are also an integral part of premature baby care. A few most notable are:

1. laboratory technicians

Laboratory technicians are responsible for running a variety of tests used to monitor and diagnose medical conditions in premature babies. From the technicians who take the X-rays to those who analyze cultures and blood samples, these medical professionals are very much involved in caring for your baby.

2. nutritionists

Nutritionists may be asked to create diets tailored to the special needs of some preemies. These people are specially trained to know the role of food components in the growth and development of a preemie.

3. pharmacists

Premature babies often require highly specialized medications in very specific doses. Your baby's physicians rely on the expertise of the hospital pharmacists to get just the right dose, and form of each prescribed medication.

4. physical therapists

Physical therapists work with preemies who need extra help with their neuromuscular development and are also involved in the follow-up developmental care of some preemies.

Chapter Three

. . . .

Medical Complications*

Because your baby was born before all of his organs and body systems were fully matured, he may have difficulty adapting to life outside the uterus.* In addition to the most common problems described in Chapter Two, some preemies also develop other complications along the road to recovery. This chapter will explain the prematurity-related problems that are most often diagnosed and treated in hospitals across America today. However, this information is given to you with a word of caution: *Do not read this chapter from beginning to end.* Don't let yourself get caught up in the kind of negative thinking that seeks out all the worst possible scenarios and imposes them on the baby. Don't use the information in this chapter to make this time more difficult than it already is.

*Some terms and medical procedures mentioned in this chapter have been explained in detail in other parts of the book, or are defined in the Glossary. Use the cross-references or the Index to find the pages that give more detailed information.

Use this chapter as you need it, one day at a time. When your baby's doctors tell you they suspect or have diagnosed a complication, look to this chapter to reinforce and expand their explanations. Use it as a resource for background information that will give you enough knowledge to ask the right questions. But remember, every preemie and every doctor create a unique circumstance of medical care. Once you know the basics, look to your baby's doctors to explain how they relate to your child's individual situation.

ANEMIA

Anemia is a medical condition caused by abnormally low concentrations of red blood cells. The actual amount of red cells babies should have depends on their chronological age and state of health; generally, newborns should have levels higher than 15 grams. When the level falls below this amount, the result is anemia. If the hemoglobin (the substance in red blood cells that carries oxygen) drops drastically below safe levels, medical intervention will be necessary.

Description

It is the job of the red blood cells to carry oxygen to all the tissues of the body. When there are not enough red blood cells to do this efficiently, a number of complications may arise. If the tissues do not get enough oxygen, their ability to function properly may be impaired. For example, the baby may exhibit problems such as poor feeding ability, poor weight gain, rapid heart rate, and/or increased caloric expenditure as he tries to compensate for the lack of oxygen. Anemia can also worsen preexisting cardiac problems by causing the heart to work harder as it tries to deliver the limited store of oxygen. Therefore, if left untreated, anemia can cause high-output congestive heart failure. Anemia can also complicate respiratory problems because the lungs may not get as much oxygen as they need. This can ultimately lead to respirator dependency.

The effects of anemia on a premature baby can range from inconsequential to very serious and even fatal. Therefore, although it is a fairly common complication of prematurity, all preemies are carefully and continuously monitored for decreasing hemoglobin levels.

Diagnosis

The diagnosis of anemia is determined by a blood test that measures the level of hemoglobin in the baby's body. This blood is drawn in small amounts either from a major blood vessel (the central method), or from the baby's heel (the capillary method), or through an umbilical catheter. A blood sample is drawn and tested at least once or twice each week until discharge. If the hemoglobin level falls below an acceptable level, the doctors will try to determine the cause so they can treat it appropriately.

These are a number of reasons why a baby may have abnormally low concentrations of hemoglobin in his blood. These reasons fall into the following two general categories:

1. in utero complications

If a baby is born anemic, it is usually due to blood loss while in the uterus. This can happen if the mother had been bleeding before delivery from complications such as placental abruption or placenta previa (page 9). It can also happen if there was a fetal-maternal hemorrhage in which the baby bled back into the placenta. Blood diverted from the fetal circulation system will leave the baby with an in-sufficient amount of red blood cells at birth.

Anemia can also result from blood incompatibility prob-lems. If, for example, the mother is Rh-negative, and the baby is Rh-positive like his father, antibodies from the moth-er can cause the baby to experience anemia. If the mother is identified as Rh-negative during her pregnancy, the problem of severe anemia can be eliminated or mini-mized by careful monitoring through blood and amniotic fluid analysis, and with the RhoGAM shots that decrease the baby's ability to form antibodies. If the mother is not given RhoGAM shots, however, each subsequent pregnancy will tend to cause more and more severe hemolysis (see Glos-sary) in each baby. When this happens, there is nothing that can be done to prevent anemia from occurring.

Another blood incompatibility problem, called ABO, may also cause hemolysis and affect the likelihood of newborn anemia. This problem develops when the mother has blood type O, and the baby has blood type A or B. Unlike Rh-factor incompatibility, there is no way to prevent ABO incompatibility from causing anemia, but the problem does not worsen with each subsequent pregnancy, and the re-sulting anemia tends to be much less critical.

Most often the in utero problems that cause an abnormal loss of red blood cells in the baby are well known to the doctors at the time of delivery. Knowing in advance that the baby may be born anemic gives them the opportunity to prepare for quick blood analysis at birth and to begin necessary treatment as soon as possible. (See the discussion of treatment later in this chapter.)

2. anemia of prematurity

All babies, premature and full-term, tend to become ane-mic at some time during the first one to three months of life. This happens because, while still in utero, the fetus does not need to be well oxygenated, and so needs a very large amount of hemoglobin to get what little oxygen he has out to the tissues of the body. After birth, however, the baby will breathe in oxygenated air and therefore won't need as much hemoglobin to get the increased levels of oxygen to the tissues of the skin, muscles, bone, and organs. Therefore, during the first few months, as the abundance of red blood cells present at birth begins to break down faster than the baby's bone marrow can produce new red blood cells, the hemoglobin level will drop and cause anemia.

This process is exaggerated in premature babies, in part because they do not get the full amount of iron (which is stored in the hemoglobin of red blood cells) that full-term babies get during the third trimester of pregnancy. This abnormally low amount of hemoglobin is then worsened as blood samples for testing are repeatedly drawn from the preemie. Since the premature baby cannot replace the lost red blood cells as quickly as they are being taken from him, anemia often results.

Anemia of prematurity also often accompanies other serious disease states. An infection, for example, can trigger the breakdown of red blood cells. Also, NEC (page 111) can cause hemorrhaging into the bowel, and an intraventricular hemorrhage (page 99) will cause bleeding into the brain cavity. These hemorrhages will cause a sudden loss of blood that may result in severe anemia requiring immediate treatment.

Treatment

The goal in treating anemia is to increase the hemoglobin level so that the body remains properly oxygenated and the body tissues suffer no damage from oxygen deprivation. That is why the baby's hemoglobin level is constantly monitored, and if it is found to be too low, its probable future course will be predicted by a careful analysis of its cause.

Sometimes, no medical treatment at all is necessary. If a preemie's hemoglobin level begins to drop at some point during the first three months of life, but he has experienced no in utero bleeding or disease complications that have caused him to lose blood, most likely his own ability to produce new red blood cells will soon mature and the anemia will resolve itself.

Some babies who experience anemia of prematurity can be treated with iron supplements. Usually, however, this is not an effective treatment until the baby is at a corrected age close to term because the younger preemie can not absorb or utilize supplemental iron, and needs not only iron but full replacement of hemoglobin. For this younger preemie red blood cells can be replaced through a blood transfusion.

Anemia in the premature infant is often treated with a blood transfusion of packed red blood cells. This blood component is different from whole blood in that it contains a higher concentration of the needed red blood cells. When a transfusion is necessary, the packed red cells are available from the hospital's blood bank, or when you know in advance that a transfusion is necessary, they can be obtained from a personally selected donor. (See "Blood Bank Information" on page 124).

A transfusion adds the red blood cells directly into the baby's total circulating blood supply. This is done through an IV or a catheter, and it takes two to three hours to complete. The procedure is completely painless except for the initial needle prick. During the transfusion, the baby will be carefully monitored for transfusion reactions such as fever, increased blood pressure or heart rate, and any change in respiration.

Transfusions may also be used to prevent anemic complications. Often babies who are already experiencing significant cardiac or respiratory problems, for example, cannot risk the additional stress of anemia. Therefore, the doctors may use transfusions to ensure that the baby's hematocrit level will stay over 15 grams (see Glossary). Then, as soon as the problem has improved, they can let the level drop to 10 grams or even lower as long as there is no evidence of an insufficient oxygen supply.

Even after a transfusion, the baby's hemoglobin level will probably drop again to below safe levels. Therefore, anemia will continue to be a problem in the premature infant until about the third month of life, when the baby can produce enough of his own red blood cells to keep the hemoglobin count at an acceptable level. Until that time, transfusions may become an ongoing part of his routine care. It is not uncommon, for example, for a very-very premature child to have ten or eleven transfusions in the first eight weeks of life.

Once the anemia is corrected and there is no indication that the baby will suffer any further unusual blood loss, you can consider the problem completely resolved. Infant anemia will have no long-term effects on the child, and it will not predispose him to becoming anemic in the future.

BRONCHOPULMONARY DYSPLASIA (BPD)

Bronchopulmonary dysplasia is a term that was first introduced in 1967 to describe changes that occur in the lungs of some infants after prolonged treatment with oxygen and mechanical ventilation. These changes include increased amounts of fluid in the lining of the lungs and cystic degeneration of the lung tissue. This causes progressive deterioration of the lung function and leads to chronic lung disease.

Although bronchopulmonary dysplasia (BPD) is occasionally found in full-term infants who have severe pulmonary problems, the disease most commonly affects premature babies with respiratory distress syndrome (RDS, page 33) who are on a respirator for more than twenty-eight days. As modern technology enables smaller and sicker preemies to survive with the aid of respirators, BPD has become one of the most common consequences of neonatal intensive care.

Because of its cyclical nature, bronchopulmonary dysplasia is especially frustrating for parents to deal with and for physicians to treat. Because preemies often have immature lungs, they need mechanical ventilation to survive. However, because of this same lung immaturity, the lungs may not be able to withstand the constant air pressure of the respirator and may begin to deteriorate. Then, even as the lungs mature, ironically, the baby cannot come off of the respirator because the damaged lungs cannot function without it. The longer the baby stays on the respirator, the more severe the degree of BPD will be, and the longer he will need the respirator. The good news is that a child with BPD who has constant and appropriate care will get better. The bad news is that the process of weaning a child from oxygen and/or respirator dependency can take several years.

Diagnosis

Any baby who requires supplemental oxygen for more than twenty-eight days is at risk for developing BPD. The diagnosis of this disease is confirmed with radiographic procedures. When BPD is present, X-rays will show evidence of fluid in the lining of the lungs, development of abnormal tissue, and a cystic degeneration of the lung tissue.

Treatment

Treatment for bronchopulmonary dysplasia actually begins as a three-step preventative procedure. Knowing the relationship between the use of a respirator and BPD, physicians will, (1) use the lowest airway pressure necessary to obtain adequate ventilation, (2) rapidly lower the pressure as the lungs improve, and (3) limit the duration of intubation as much by trying to get the baby to nasal CPAP or an oxygen hood as soon as possible. These three steps alone can eliminate or minimize the occurrence of BPD. However, once BPD is evident, corrective treatment is necessary.

The goal in treating BPD is to maintain all vital signs while slowly weaning the baby from the respirator. Constant and consistent nursing and medical care are the keys to doing this effectively. To begin, the baby's doctors and nurses will diligently administer chest physiotherapy and suctioning. They may also try to reduce environmental stimulation around the baby. Many preemies are very sensitive to light, sound, and touch, and may respond with changes in heart and breathing rates when overstimulated. These changes can complicate recovery from BPD, so you may be asked to let your baby lie quiet and undisturbed. Then, the baby may be given medications that can help lessen the effects of the initial lung damage and make it possible for him to be cared for at home. These medications include bronchodilators like theophylline that open the bronchial tubes and make breathing less strenuous. Inhalation treatments are also used to overcome bronchospasms. Babies with BPD will be given diuretics, such as Lasix, to reduce the amount of fluid collecting in the lungs. These babies can't tolerate excessive or sometimes even normal amounts of fluid. So in addition to the medication, the doctors will limit their water and salt intake to the minimum required to provide necessary calories for metabolic needs and growth.

Babies with BPD often cannot tolerate breast or bottle feedings, and yet need an exceptionally high number of calories to support the energy they expend struggling to breathe. This, combined with the restricted fluid intake, can affect the baby's growth, and his ability to recover from the lung disease. Therefore, as part of the treatment for BPD, a baby is often fed a highly concentrated solution of total parenteral nutrition (page 38) through a catheter (page 39), and then begins his early oral feedings through an NG tube (page 42).

Throughout the treatment period, the doctors will continue their efforts to wean the baby from the respirator. They will constantly monitor the arterial blood gases as they gradually reduce the pressure and oxygen rate. This weaning process can take anywhere from a few weeks to several months. Finally, when the baby is able to maintain acceptable blood gas levels for twenty-four hours or longer while on continuous positive air pressure (CPAP, page 35), the doctors may attempt to remove him from the respirator. If, after an extended period of time, a baby cannot be safely removed from the respirator, it may be necessary to surgically insert a tracheostomy tube. This tube will allow direct ventilation through the trachea while leaving the mouth and nose free of respiratory apparatus.

When a BPD baby can be safely taken off the respirator, he will still need continuous attention to overcome its effects. He will continue with the frequent chest physiotherapy and suctioning, which prevent airway obstruction and lung collapse that result from secretions remaining in the lungs. Some of these babies also need oxygen therapy for several months or even years to assure adequate oxygenation of the body's tissues and to avoid pulmonary hypertension and the complications associated with chronically low oxygen levels. This supplemental oxygen can be delivered to the baby through an oxygen hood or tent, or with a face mask, or through a nasal catheter or cannula. Although this need for oxygen therapy prolongs the baby's hospital stay, increasing numbers of babies can now eventually receive their oxygen therapy at home. This, of course, is a better environment in which the baby can grow and bond with his parents and siblings; it also reduces the financial burden of extended hospital care.

Little is known about the long-term evolution of BPD. However, it is known, that, with well-supervised and supported home care the vast majority of BPD preemies show progressive improvement and eventually do recover from the effects of the disease; almost all are weaned from supplemental oxygen sometime in the first two years of life. Many of these children will be readmitted to the hospital during the first year because they are prone to pulmonary problems such as pneumonia, other respiratory tract infections, and airway obstruction. But even the occurrence of these readmissions is becoming less frequent as parents and health care providers become more adept at caring for BPD babies at home.

The future holds exciting possibilities for the prevention and treatment of BPD. Already research and clinical studies with animals have found that, when an experimental surfactant replacement (see Glossary) is introduced into the trachea right after birth, the incidence and severity of respiratory distress syndrome (and therefore BPD) is dramatically decreased. It's also now known that the risk of BPD may be minimized by changing the ventilating pattern of the respirator. Respirators usually control a baby's breathing rate at somewhere between 30 and 60 breaths per minute. Theoretically, new high-frequency ventilation (HFV) could manage a baby's breathing at 500 to 2000 breaths per minute. Rather than moving the baby's chest in the customary in-out regulated pace, the HFV would drastically increase the rate of breathing, thereby reducing the pressure on the lungs.

For now, it is comforting to know that a child with BPD will get better, and that administration of oxygen at home is a manageable reality of today's preemie care. See "David's Story" on page 166 for more details on home care management.

INFECTIONS

Infections occur when organisms such as bacteria, viruses, and other agents enter the body and change the stability of the vital signs (respiration and heart rate, body temperature, and skin color). Premature babies are especially prone to infection because their antibody (an infection-fighting element in the blood) level is insufficient to fight off invading infectious agents. Infections commonly found in premature infants include pneumonia, sepsis, and meningitis. Each of these is explained in detail below.

There are a number of ways a baby may develop an infection. Infections like pneumonia, sepsis, and meningitis very often develop from Group B Strep (GBS) infections (or less frequently from *E. coli, Listeria,* and other forms of bacteria) that the baby can pick up from the mother during the birthing process. She, herself, may have no symptoms or problems from this infection, but because it is present in her vaginal tract, it can easily be passed on to the baby if he swallows fluids during birth.

Sometimes these infections may be bacteremic, which means they get into the blood but give no symptoms and may not need prolonged, intensive treatment. Other times they are septic, meaning that once the bacteria are in the blood, the babies show symptoms of infection and need immediate treatment. Because many women have Group B Strep as a normal part of their vaginal flora without any symptoms or suspect conditions, the birth of an infected baby is unexpected and therefore diagnosis and treatment may be delayed. Other babies, however, are at risk for developing Group B Strep infections because their mothers had ruptured membranes (page 10) 24 to 48 hours or more before the actual birth, or had a high fever at the time of birth, or showed evidence of a placental infection called chorioamnionitis. These at-risk babies will receive immediate treatment even before a confirming laboratory diagnosis is made. (This is especially true when cultures are used because they take at least two to three days to grow before they can be analyzed.) The sooner treatment is begun, the more likely it is that the infection will not progress to an advanced stage.

Some premature babies acquire bacterial infections directly from the hospital environment in which they live; these are called nosocomial infections. Contrary to popular belief, hospitals are not sterile places. Although you may wash your hands and wear a hospital gown over your clothing when you visit your baby, this doesn't make you completely germ free. And although the nursery personnel also will scrub, sterilize equipment, and use masks and gloves when necessary, it is impossible to completely eliminate the presence of bacteria. Most environmental bacteria are totally harmless as they colonize on the skin's surface. However, Group B Strep infections, along with *Staphylococcus aureus* and *Staphylococcus epidermidis* infections, can find their way into the baby's body at any point where there is a breakdown in the skin's surface. These entry points include all the insertion sites of IVs, catheters, respiratory and feeding tubes, and any surgical incisions. There are also several kinds of bacteria called gram-negative organisms that thrive in water and that may find their way into the respiratory system, through the respiratory equipment, and cause pneumonia. Obviously, the smaller the baby, and the more medical intervention that is necessary, the more likely is the occurrence of a hospital-acquired infection.

One technique of infection control is isolation of the infected infant. If the doctors suspect that your baby has a communicable infection, you may find him removed from the nursery area. He may be put in another room, or another unit in the hospital, or simply moved to an isolated area of the nursery.

These nosocomial infections are the most common cause

of death in premature infants after the first week of life. This is an alarming fact, but it is the price of advanced technology and is often unavoidable in crowded intensive care nurseries that are treating many very small preemies who need extensive invasive treatment. The physicians caring for these babies realize that by inserting tubes, catheters, and needles into them, they are risking infectious exposure, but they also know that if they don't proceed with the necessary treatment, they are jeopardizing the babies' chances for survival. The very same technological advancements that give unprecedented hope to the families of premature babies carry with them the risk of infection and death. Despite this, the fact remains that approximately 95 percent of all premature babies born in the United States today will survive.

Pneumonia

Pneumonia is an infection in the area of the lung involved in the exchange of carbon dioxide and oxygen. The inflammation reduces the amount of space available for the exchange of air and therefore interferes with adequate oxygenation of the body. Pneumonia, therefore, compounds any of the other prematurity-related respiratory problems (page 33).

The symptoms of pneumonia include a change in the breathing rate or pattern, difficulty in breathing, and increased episodes of apnea (page 31). The diagnosis is based on clinical observations of these symptoms as well as the detection of the sound of fluid in the lungs. Diagnosis is confirmed with blood tests, by X-rays of the lungs, and/or with cultures taken by inserting a tube into the lung and obtaining a sample of the lung fluid.

The primary treatment for pneumonia is a one- to three-week course of antibiotics. These antibiotics are given on a prescribed schedule through an IV or by injection. In addition, support measures are taken to maintain the baby's vital signs. He may need supplemental oxygen (page 34) or intubation (page 35) for efficient exchange of oxygen and carbon dioxide.

When pneumonia is diagnosed early and treated quickly, the baby has an excellent chance of complete recovery. However, if left undetected or untreated for too long, pneumonia can become a deadly infection or lead to sepsis or meningitis.

Sepsis

Sepsis is a medical condition in which there is bacteria in the bloodstream. The bacteria travel in the blood to many parts of the body and cause notable changes in the baby's health. These changes can be subtle or catastrophic. A doctor or nurse may notice that the baby's skin color or his feeding ability is not as good as it was the day before. Or, the baby may have an increased incidence of apnea episodes (page 31). Diagnosis is usually made with a blood culture and other blood tests.

Sepsis often brings infection to the lungs and therefore may accompany a bout of pneumonia. The treatment for sepsis is the same as that for pneumonia: antibiotics given for one to three weeks through IV or injection. In addition, the baby's vital signs are supported, with special attention paid to his blood pressure, which can be stabilized with an infusion of blood or plasma, or with medications such as vasopressors like dopamine and epinephrine.

Very often these measures will effectively combat sepsis and the baby will recover without any ill effects. But because sepsis brings infection to all parts of the body through the bloodstream, sometimes the preemie can't handle the extensive invasion and the infection will be fatal.

Meningitis

Meningitis is an infection or inflammation of the spinal cord and the lining of the layers around the brain. The doctors will suspect that a baby has meningitis if his perinatal medical history indicates that his mother may have been infected or if the baby's clinical condition is significantly affected. The baby may show evidence of changing stability in vital signs, poor weight gain, and increased episodes of apnea (page 31). To diagnose meningitis, the doctors will order a spinal tap.

A spinal tap is performed in the nursery. To protect the baby from further infection, the doctors will wear masks and gloves, and will drape off the area. The baby will be placed on his side and curled in the fetal position. The area of the proposed needle injection will be prepared with an antiseptic solution. Then, a short, narrow needle is inserted between two lumbar vertebrae into the area where there is spinal fluid (not into the spinal cord itself). A sample of the fluid is withdrawn for analysis and the spinal tap is completed with virtually no risk of disability. Anesthesia is generally not used for this procedure for two reasons. First, the initial prick of the needle used to administer the anesthesia is equal to the discomfort of the prick of the spinal tap needle itself. Secondly, the swelling caused by anesthesia can obscure the vertebrae, making the procedure more difficult than necessary.

Treatment for meningitis is similar to that for pneumonia and sepsis, but because some antibiotics cannot pass into the spinal fluid, the antibiotic may be a different type and dosage, and is usually given for a longer period of time (two to three weeks). The baby's vital signs will be supported during treatment, and once the diagnosis of meningitis has been confirmed (remember that treatment may begin in infants at risk before the results of all the diagnostic tests are available), the baby may need more intensive care. Because meningitis irritates the brain structure and causes changes in the blood supply to the brain, radiographic evaluations such as ultrasounds, computerized axial tomography scans, and magnetic resonance imaging (MRI) may be used to monitor potential damage to the brain. As part of this monitoring process, a pediatric neurologist (page 71) may be called in to perform regular neurological examinations. Then, prior to discharge, an audiologist (page 69) may also be asked to evaluate the baby's hearing because meningitis has been found to cause some cases of hearing impairment.

The outcome and long-term effects of meningitis depend on what kind of complications were involved in the early stages of the infection. If the baby experienced seizures, coma, or a poor response to treatment, the infection may lead to brain damage, or even death. If the infection was diagnosed and treated before progressing to advanced stages, the baby should recover with no long-term effects at all.

Other Infections

Premature babies are also prone to other infections, such as skin and urinary tract infections. These kinds of infection are less serious than sepsis, pneumonia, or meningitis, and are usually diagnosed and treated easily, without great worry or concern. However, it is often the case in premature baby care that medical complications are interrelated. The treatment for one may cause another; the aftereffects of a corrected condition may lead to the start of something else; and so on. This ongoing trail of possible complications caused by other complications is unpredictable and further emphasizes the need to parent a premature baby one day at a time.

INTRAVENTRICULAR HEMORRHAGE (IVH)

An intraventricular hemorrhage or IVH (sometimes also called an intracranial hemorrhage or a brain bleed) is a medical condition that results from abnormal bleeding on the surface of the brain, in the substance of the brain, or in the brain's central chambers (called ventricles) that are continuous with the canal of the spinal cord. The vast majority of these brain bleeds occur in the very first week of life; after that time, it is very unlikely that one will occur. For some babies (especially those born at less than 34 weeks gestational age and/or weighing less than 3 pounds 5 ounces), IVH is an unavoidable consequence of premature birth.

Description

The exact cause of intraventricular hemorrhage has been the controversial subject of many studies. However, it is generally believed that the immature and fragile blood vessels in and around the preemie's brain are prone to rupture if the baby experiences fluctuations in blood pressure or when the brain is insufficiently oxygenated. Unlike full-term babies (who very rarely have IVH), premature babies have not yet developed the protective mechanism that automatically preserves sufficient and consistent blood flow into the brain in the event of changing blood pressure or oxygen supply. It has also been found that the smaller babies, who are by nature more likely to experience asphyxia, respiratory distress syndrome, or other pulmonary diseases that put stress on the brain's circulatory system, are at increased risk for having ruptured blood vessels in the brain.

Intraventricular hemorrhages are categorized into four different degrees or grades of severity:

• A grade 1 bleed is the mildest degree of hemorrhage. It is a hemorrhage in which a small amount of blood is found in the area of the brain that has a lot of blood vessels and grows rapidly during fetal life. (Sometimes this grade is even subdivided into a grade 0 bleed, called a subarachnoid hemorrhage, in which a small amount of blood is found on the outer surface of the brain.)

• A grade 2 bleed is a hemorrhage in which a small amount of blood is found inside the brain ventricles, but the excess blood doesn't cause the ventricles to enlarge.

• A grade 3 bleed is a hemorrhage in which a greater volume of blood is found in the brain ventricles, causing the ventricles to enlarge, but often only temporarily.

• A grade 4 bleed is the most severe degree of IVH, in which blood is found in the brain substance itself.

Diagnosis

A preemie's physicians are always alert to the observable signs of an intraventricular hemorrhage. These symptoms include: a worsening respiratory disease, a rapidly enlarging head, vomiting, irritability, lethargy, abnormal eye signs (glazed, rolling, or staring eyes), an abnormal neurological exam (perhaps as determined in consultation with a pediatric neurologist, page 71), and/or seizures. If the hemorrhage has been fairly extensive, a large amount of blood will leave the circulatory system as it bleeds into the brain area. This can cause a drop in red blood cell levels and the onset of anemia and/or jaundice. On the other hand, the lesser-grade hemorrhage may be "silent" without any observable signs.

Ultrasonography is the best and most reliable technique for diagnosing intraventricular hemorrhage. It is a sensitive, extremely accurate, painless, and relatively inexpensive method of diagnosis that is done without the use of radiation. Also, ultrasound scans (also called sonograms) are a desirable means of assessing IVH because they are performed right in the nursery with minimal handling of the baby. This eliminates the potential risk involved in transporting a small, sick preemie to another area of the hospital. During the examination, a transducer is placed on the front of the head over the baby's soft spot (the area of the brain where the skull bones have not yet grown together, called the anterior fontanelle). The technician slowly scans the area and images of the brain are recorded on a videotape that is later analyzed by the neonatologist and a pediatric radiologist (page 77). Sometimes these results will pinpoint the exact degree of the blood in the affected area and will give the physicians the information they need to determine appropriate treatment.

Other times the ultrasound will indicate a possible bleed, but will not give conclusive information. In these cases the doctors will often do a spinal tap. In this procedure, a small needle is inserted between two vertebrae in the spinal column. Fluid is then withdrawn. If blood and certain other chemical values are present in the fluid, IVH is confirmed and treatment will begin.

Treatment

Once intraventricular hemorrhage has been diagnosed, the first order of treatment is vigilant monitoring. Weekly ultrasound scans will be performed to watch the progression of the bleed. The baby's head circumference will be measured regularly to watch for the kind of rapid growth that would indicate enlargement of the ventricles. Also, doctors and nurses will continually observe the baby for any signs of worsening respiratory or pulmonary conditions. During this time, the neonatologist may call in a pediatric neurologist (page 71), who will examine the baby for any signs of developmental problems that can be caused by the change in blood flow to the brain.

If a preemie has a grade 1 bleed, it is very unlikely that he will need any treatment at all. Most often the body reabsorbs the hemorrhaged blood within two to three weeks after the bleed. The baby's chances of developing any developmental handicaps are the same as if no hemorrhage at all had occurred.

There is great variability in the treatment of grade 2 and grade 3 hemorrhages. Twenty-five percent of these bleeds will not cause any ventricular enlargement, will subside by themselves, and therefore will not need any medical intervention. Other times, although the grade 2 or grade 3 bleed does cause ventricle enlargement, the enlargement is slight and does not increase the circumference of the child's head more than 1 to 2 centimeters per week (which is normal growth). In these cases, again, the bleed stops by itself and the ventricles return to normal size within the first year without any treatment. However, if the ventricle continues to enlarge, causing increasing pressure on the brain, the baby may be given medications that can decrease the size of the enlarged ventricle and inhibit the production of cerebrospinal fluid. This reduces the pressure on the brain and lessens the chance of long-term neurological problems. Research reports predict that up to 25 percent of grade 2 and grade 3 hemorrhages will progress to a complication called hydrocephalus and will require surgery (as described later). However, many hospitals are now finding that this figure is actually smaller than five percent, which is encouraging news.

A grade 4 hemorrhage usually needs more intensive treatment because it can damage the tissues of the brain. As the hemorrhage flows into the substance of the brain, it settles in newly created pockets. As the blood is reabsorbed into the body, these pockets remain as holes in the brain tissue (these are called porencephalic cysts). If these holes are coupled with the enlarged ventricle of a grade 3 hemorrhage, there may be an obstruction of the normal flow of spinal fluid. This can cause hydrocephalus, which is characterized by an abnormal increase in head size and a progressive loss of brain tissue. Sometimes hydrocephalus must be surgically treated.

If the baby's head size continues to enlarge without any relief in the pressure on the brain tissues, a surgical procedure to put in a ventriculoperitoneal shunt will be performed by a pediatric neurosurgeon. This shunt is a tube that provides an alternate mechanism for removing the fluid trapped in the ventricles by the obstructed spinal fluid pathways. The tube is surgically inserted into the side of the head, through the brain, and into the ventricle. The other end of the tube is threaded beneath the surface of the skin behind the ear and down into the abdominal area, where the fluid can drain and be reabsorbed by the body. With the shunt in place and working, the ventricle most often returns to normal size. Although some children will outgrow the need for this drainage tube, many will need it for life. This is not as cumbersome as it sounds. When the child develops more fat layers and grows more hair there is no visible evidence of the shunt, and it does not cause the child any discomfort or inconvenience.

At the point where hydrocephalus requires shunting, abnormal neurological development becomes a significant possibility. Because grade 4 hemorrhages can cause changes in the brain's metabolism and blood flow, and can do physical damage to the brain itself, approximately 50 percent of these babies will have significant long-term developmental problems. These problems can include seizures, motor problems, low intelligence level, blindness, speech and/or hearing impairment, and/or cerebral palsy.

It would be misleading to suggest that there is an absolute relationship between brain hemorrhage and neurological outcome. There are many preemies who have had severe grade 4 hemorrhages without suffering any neurological impairment. There are also babies who have had no IVH and yet have severe developmental problems. It appears from clinical evidence that changes in the blood supply to the brain can severely handicap some preemies and leave others unscathed.

Medical researchers may still have a lot to learn about the long-term effects of intraventricular hemorrhages, but today's premature babies have a distinct advantage over those born just a few years ago. In the early 1980s between 39 and 58 percent of all babies born before 34 weeks gestational age developed IVH. Today's studies find that these numbers are definitely decreasing. It is unclear whether this is due to better methods of diagnosis, treatment applications, general handling techniques, or improved professional training. But the fact is: Fewer premature babies are developing IVH. Also, early diagnosis with an ultrasound scan and the availability of immediate treatment can be credited with drastically reducing the number of cases in which an IVH leads to a catastrophic outcome. Until very recently, an IVH was diagnosed and monitored with computed tomographic (CT) scans. These scans were not as accurate or specific as ultrasound scans (especially when looking for lower-grade bleeds), and they could not be performed in the nursery. This made it necessary to jeopardize the baby's stability by removing him from his secure environment and transporting him to the radiology unit.

Although not as efficient as ultrasound, a CT scan was far better than the previous method of diagnosis. Until the early 1970s, most intraventricular hemorrhages were diagnosed at the time of autopsy. Without any means of seeing into the brain, physicians could not detect silent or low-grade bleeds, and could not intervene to prevent the progression to obstructive hydrocephalus. Today, thanks to improvements in modern technology, the occurrence of an IVH does not go undiagnosed or untreated when treatment is necessary. Now, an IVH does not automatically mean death or a handicapped existence for the child.

Perhaps tomorrow medical science will find a way to eliminate or lessen the effects of intraventricular hemorrhages. This could happen when we find a way to help the preemie self-regulate a consistent flow of blood to the brain; or maybe there will be a way to strengthen the fragile blood vessels of the brain that are so easily ruptured in the first few days after birth. It's also possible that continued studies with positron emission tomography (PET) will enable researchers to document changes in the cerebral metabolism that will show them how to preserve neurological development by preventing changes at the cellular level that may predispose certain babies to hemorrhage, or others to have handicaps even without having suffered a hemorrhage. The future promises untold medical improvements in the care of preemies prone to brain hemorrhages.

For now, however, some preemies do get intraventricular hemorrhages; some will suffer neurological impairment, and some will die. But the number of these cases is decreasing every day. If your baby has an IVH, the recent advances in medical science offer you unprecedented hope for a positive outcome.

JAUNDICE

Jaundice (also called hyperbilirubinemia) is fairly common among all newborns and is not usually a serious condition. It occurs when there is an overabundance of bilirubin in the body. Bilirubin is a yellowish red pigment found in small amounts in everyone's blood. Normally, bilirubin is released into the bloodstream during the breakdown of red blood cells. Then it binds to protein molecules that transport it to the liver, where it is metabolized and then expelled from the body through the intestinal tract. However, sometimes excess amounts of bilirubin will be produced in a baby's body, causing him to develop jaundice.

Babies are particularly prone to jaundice for a number of reasons. All babies have an extra amount of red blood cells at birth; this leads to a rapid increase in the breakdown of red blood cells and therefore the amount of bilirubin in the body. A baby's liver may not be fully developed enough to process this large amount of bilirubin. Infants also have lower levels of protein for the bilirubin to adhere to and use as transport to the liver. Therefore, a larger than normal amount will stay in the body.

Although jaundice is common in newborns and is often harmless, it cannot be ignored. As the levels of bilirubin build up in the body, they will seep through the tissues of the skin, causing a yellowing of the skin and the whites of the eyes. If the bilirubin level continues to go up, it may pass through the blood/brain barrier causing irreversible brain damage. This extreme complication of jaundice is called bilirubin encephalopathy or kernicterus. This is a rare occurrence and it is very difficult to predict at what level of bilirubin the baby's health status changes from simple jaundice to kernicterus.

Diagnosis

A premature baby is more likely to develop jaundice than a full-term baby because his liver is more likely to be underdeveloped, he has lower levels of blood protein, and since many preemies do not have oral feedings in the first few days of life, the bilirubin does not have full opportunity to exit through bowel movements. Knowing this, the baby's doctor will take several prophylactic measures to ensure that the level of bilirubin in the baby's blood does not reach concentrations high enough to do damage to the central nervous system.

A preemie's bilirubin level will peak sometime between the fifth and seventh day of life. During this time, his nurses and doctors will observe him closely for signs of yellowing, and blood samples will be taken (usually from his heel) to monitor the levels of bilirubin. The blood test results will rate the bilirubin level on a numbered scale—the higher the number, the higher the level of bilirubin. This numbered score will aid the doctor in determining appropriate treatment.

The exact number at which a child is susceptible to kernicterus is unknown. It appears that the more premature the baby, the lower the level of bilirubin that may be dangerous. Therefore it is impossible to set an exact number and say, "Any child with a bilirubin count over this number should receive medical treatment." The decision to begin treatment for jaundice depends on the significance of the bilirubin level relative to the baby's age, weight, and state of general health. This is why it could happen that your baby, with a bilirubin score of 12, will not receive any treatment at all, and yet your sister's baby with the same score will receive intensive medical therapy.

The following *general* guidelines will give you an idea of how physicians determine which babies with jaundice should be medically treated and which should be left alone to allow the liver to develop and process the excess bilirubin without medical intervention:

• Full-term babies are generally safe with bilirubin levels below 20.
• A moderately premature baby (one born at 35 to 37 weeks gestation with a weight of between 3 pounds 12 ounces and 7 pounds 8 ounces) is generally safe with bilirubin levels below 15 to 18.
• A very premature baby (one born at 30 to 34 weeks gestation with a weight of between 2 pounds 3 ounces and

5 pounds 8 ounces) is generally safe with bilirubin levels below 12 to 15.

• A very-very premature baby (one born at 25 to 29 weeks gestation with a weight of between 1 pound 5 ounces and 3 pounds 8½ ounces) is generally safe with bilirubin levels below 10 to 12.

If a baby's bilirubin count comes within three to five points of the top level of his safety zone, his physician may begin treatment to avoid the possible complications of going over that inexact danger point.

Treatment

The first mode of treatment is a procedure called phototherapy. This is a painless process in which the child is placed under special fluorescent lights that can break down the structure of the bilirubin in the tissues of the skin so it can be more easily transported to the liver and then excreted from the body. These lights now come in a variety of colors, each having varying wave length characteristics. The newest light is "superblue," and it has very specific light characteristics to provide a faster breakdown of the bilirubin.

Phototherapy (also called bililight treatment) is a simple procedure that is performed right in the nursery. The lights are placed above or alongside the baby's incubator, or may be built right into the lighting system of a radiant warmer. The lights are left on around the clock, but the nurses will usually turn them off when you visit your baby so the treatments won't interfere with your time together. The baby is usually kept naked (except perhaps for a diaper), and his position is changed periodically to give his full body surface the benefit of the treatment. His eyes are masked to shield them from the lights, and all his monitoring wires remain in place. His feeding schedule continues as before, but some babies are temporarily taken off breast milk during this treatment period because in a very small number of cases breast milk can actually raise the bilirubin count. (If your baby is taken off your breast milk, be sure to pump and store your milk during this time.) During the treatment period you may notice that your baby's stools are very loose and sometimes greenish in color. He may need IV fluids to prevent dehydration. He may also sleep more than usual, and develop a slight rash. These are common reactions to the bililights and will disappear as soon as the treatments are discontinued.

Phototherapy treatments generally are given for three to ten days until blood samples indicate the amount of bilirubin in the body has decreased to a safe level. When the treatments are discontinued there may be a rebound effect that causes the bilirubin count to go back up, but it will quickly drop down again. Most often phototherapy treatments are entirely successful.

However, occasionally an elevated bilirubin count will persist. When this happens the doctors will continue the phototherapy and look for underlying causes. These can include metabolic imbalances such as low thyroid disease, a blockage in the intestinal tract that is slowing the passage of stools and the exit of the bilirubin, and/or conditions such as Rh or ABO incompatibilities (page 85) or sepsis (page 96), all of which can affect the breakdown of red blood cells. When the underlying cause is diagnosed and treated, the bilirubin count most often decreases.

Since phototherapy appears so simple and painless, you may wonder why it isn't given to all preemies just as a precautionary measure. Physicians will carefully monitor the results of the bilirubin blood tests and give phototherapy treatments only when absolutely necessary because it has possible negative side effects. These include skin rashes, potential eye problems, diarrhea, sweating, dehydration, and weight loss. These side effects may interfere with the baby's ability to grow and thrive.

Sometimes, right from the start or despite phototherapy, the bilirubin count is too high to be properly treated with the introduction or the continuance of phototherapy. To protect the baby from possible kernicterus, his attending physician may give him an exchange transfusion. At what point the bilirubin count is too high is an arbitrary decision made by the doctor. A general rule of thumb says "too" high is the point at which there is one milligram of bilirubin per hundred grams of body weight. Using this formula, a 1000-gram baby will have a transfusion when his bili count goes over 10; a 1500-gram baby will have a transfusion when his bili count goes over 15; a 2000-gram baby will have a transfusion when his bili count goes over 20. For babies who weigh less than 1000 grams, the doctor will probably wait until the count reaches 10 before performing a transfusion.

An exchange transfusion is done right in the nursery by the attending physician. The baby is left on the radiant warmer or in his incubator, and it takes one to two hours to complete. In this kind of transfusion small amounts of the baby's blood are slowly withdrawn and then replaced with equal amounts of donor blood. This can be done by any one of three methods:

1. If the baby already has two umbilical catheters in place for other medical purposes (page 39), the transfusion can be given through these. The baby's blood is withdrawn from one catheter while donor blood is given through the other. With this method of even exchange, there is no change in the baby's blood volume, which avoids the complication of putting undue stress on his heart.

2. An umbilical catheter with a three-way stopcock can be placed into a vein. The bilirubin is exchanged in a three-step procedure: a small amount of blood (perhaps 10 cubic centimeters) is withdrawn from the baby. The stopcock is closed to the baby and opened to discard the blood into a

collection bag. The stopcock is then opened so the same amount of donor blood can be inserted into the vein. This procedure is repeated over and over again until twice the baby's blood volume has been exchanged.

3. The exchange transfusion can be given through a peripheral vein and artery. Donor blood is usually transfused into the vein, and the baby's blood is drawn from the artery. Because the baby's veins are so small, this is the most difficult method to use.

Whichever method your baby's doctors choose, there is the possibility that the bilirubin count won't go down to safe levels after the first transfusion. Some babies will need several transfusions before the count can be brought under control.

Like phototherapy, exchange transfusions will be given only when absolutely necessary. Although considered a safe and sometimes routine procedure, there is always a potential for transfusion-reaction complications. Anyone who receives a blood transfusion risks the hazards of mismatched blood, mechanical problems, contamination of equipment, infection, and the transmission of infectious diseases such as hepatitis, syphilis, or AIDS. If your baby needs a transfusion, you can decrease some of the potential risks by using a designated donor. Read "Blood Bank Information" on page 124 and talk to your baby's doctor about this.

Once the bilirubin count has been brought down to an acceptable level, the baby's liver will be able to process it without further problems. Jaundice in infancy leaves no lasting effects on the baby.

NECROTIZING ENTEROCOLITIS (NEC)

Necrotizing enterocolitis is an illness that is characterized by a deterioration of the intestinal tract. The problem very often stems from an abnormal or obstructed flow of blood to the intestines, which allows abnormal bacterial activity to colonize the gastointestinal tract. This may eventually cause infection, and the bacteria may produce gas bubbles that further disrupt its function. If left untreated, the infection may spread throughout the abdominal cavity and cause death. Although this disease is also found in full-term babies, 80 percent of the cases involve preemies weighing less than 5 pounds 8 ounces. (There are approximately three thousand to six thousand cases each year in the United States.)

In addition to a preemie's immature GI tract, there are many underlying factors that may cause an infant to develop NEC, but no single causative factor has yet been isolated. It is clear that the infants at highest risk for developing this disease are those with other significant perinatal complications that affect the flow of blood, such as fetal asphyxia (which may be caused by cord compression, placental abruption, or fetal-maternal hemorrhage), frequent episodes of apnea, bradycardia, or sepsis. These at-risk babies are carefully watched for any symptoms of NEC, which include temperature instability, lethargy, poor feeding, abdominal distension, blood in the stools, or vomiting of bile, blood, or even milk. These symptoms are sometimes accompanied by increased episodes of apnea and bradycardia, and may progress to shock, intestinal perforation, and gangrene of the bowel.

Diagnosis

Diagnosis of NEC begins with careful observation of high-risk infants for any of the previously mentioned symptoms. Babies suspected of having NEC will undergo a series of safe and painless diagnostic procedures that include

1. serial X-rays of the abdominal area to check for air

pockets in the intestinal walls, and for distention or perforation of the bowel.

2. bacterial cultures, which will be grown from stool,
blood, and throat samples.

3. blood samples (usually drawn from the baby's heel) to
check for elevated amounts of white blood cells.

4. blood gas analysis to measure the amount of acid in
the blood.

If these diagnostic procedures indicate the presence of
NEC, treatments will begin immediately.

Treatment

Once NEC has been diagnosed, the physician will discontinue the baby's oral feedings. This will give the bowel a
chance to rest by reducing the amount of waste it must
process. During this time the baby will be nourished with
IV fluids. If the oral feedings are discontinued for more
than three or four days, the child may be given total parenteral nutrition (also called hyperalimentation) to meet his
caloric and nutritional needs.

The second method of treatment involves the decom-
pression of the GI tract. This is done by threading a tube
down through the baby's mouth to his stomach and suctioning out air and the contents of the stomach. This will
reduce the chance of bowel perforation and will ease the
baby's pain and make him more comfortable.

During the treatment period the baby's abdomen will
be continually X-rayed (often every 4 to 8 hours) and his
blood will be analyzed to monitor the progression of the
disease.

If the culture results indicate that NEC has an associated
infection, antibiotics will be given either intravenously or
through a tube directly into the GI tract. Oral feedings
will be reinstituted when the antibiotic course is com-

pleted (usually within seven to fourteen days) and the radiographic appearance of the bowel is normal. These feedings will begin with clear fluids for one to two days, and then will gradually be switched to formula or breast milk.

The response to this treatment is varied. NEC will recur in about 10 percent of the cases. When this happens the course of treatment described above will be repeated. With early and consistent management, 75 percent of the babies with NEC will respond favorably. Sometimes NEC leaves the baby with colonic strictures that cause a narrowing of the bowel. Usually this condition improves by itself with time, but when it doesn't, the baby may need surgery to repair the bowel. In a small percentage of babies, medical therapy may be unsuccessful and surgery will be necessary to remove the diseased part of the intestinal tract and rejoin the healthy ends of the intestines. If a large portion of the intestine is surgically removed, the baby may require a temporary ileostomy or colostomy. The healthy end of the intestine is brought through the abdominal wall and the digestive tract empties its waste through the opening in the abdominal wall into a bag. This will give the part of the intestinal tract left inside the body a chance to rest and grow. Six months to a year later, the two healthy ends of the intestinal tract will be rejoined and the child will have a fully functioning intestinal tract.

There is a 30 percent chance of death if NEC progresses to an advanced stage where it is accompanied by a gastrointestinal hemorrhage and/or septic shock. (This is a body infection that causes a drop in the stability of vital signs and blood pressure due to a decrease in heart functioning.) This statistic is not as alarming as it first sounds, however, because with early diagnosis, quick treatment, and the use of new surgical techniques, there is virtually no danger of death. Today, very few cases of NEC progress to the advanced stage.

PATENT DUCTUS ARTERIOSUS (PDA)

Patent ductus arteriosus (PDA), one of the cardiac disorders most common to premature babies, is a condition in which the blood vessel that connects the aorta (the main artery of the body) and the pulmonary artery (the artery that brings blood to the lungs) does not close as it should shortly after birth.

Description

In fetal life, the PDA blood vessel absolutely must be open so that oxygenated blood cells can travel in large quantities to the lungs. Since the fetus does not breathe oxygenated air while in utero, it is vital that excessive amounts of oxygen-carrying blood be shunted (directed) from the high pressure system in the pulmonary artery to the low pressure system in the aorta; this is called a right-to-left shunt. If the PDA were not open, the fetus would die of acute heart failure in utero, or he would develop serious pulmonary hypertension and could die shortly after birth.

At birth the PDA in all babies is still open. As the pressure in the pulmonary artery goes down when the baby starts to breathe on his own and the lungs begin to expand, there are a variety of natural chemicals in the body that will cause the PDA to close spontaneously. In full-term babies this will usually happen sometime during the first week of life, but in preemies the ductus may remain open for one to three months, depending on the maturity of the baby, the degree of respiratory problems encountered, how well oxygenated the baby is, and the levels of certain prostaglandins.

Some babies will not suffer from a lack of oxygen while the PDA is open and therefore will not require treatment. Because the open PDA over-circulates the lungs with blood, however, it becomes a potential cause of severe complica-

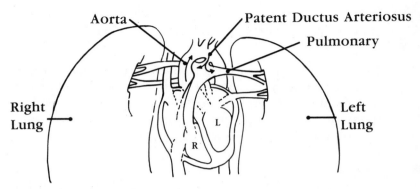

Patent Ductus Arteriosus

tions in some babies (especially the very-very premature and/or critically ill infant). These complications include medical conditions such as congestive heart failure, necrotizing enterocolitis (page 111), pulmonary edema (fluid on the lungs), and oxygen and/or respirator dependency. Therefore, although PDA is a natural birth occurrence that will ultimately correct itself, in the premature infant it will very often require treatment to avoid progressive complications that would prolong the need for intensive hospital care.

Diagnosis

The diagnosis of PDA is usually made by a neonatologist in consultation with a pediatric cardiologist (page 75). Doctors will suspect an open ductus if, through a stethoscope, they hear the sound of abnormal blood flow in the rhythmic expansion and contraction cycles of the heart. This is called a continuous murmur. Some babies, however, have a "silent" ductus in which the abnormal blood flow can not be heard, and so doctors will also use clinical observation to diagnose PDA. If a baby appears to be well oxygenated and has good skin coloring, but has difficulty breathing when taken off the respirator, this can indicate the presence of PDA. Also, because the PDA causes a left-to-right shunt in the blood flow after birth, the blood pressure will become a bit wide; this means that instead of being 60/40, for example, it might be 70/20. This widening between the two numbers of the blood pressure reading occurs because the blood is running off from the aorta through the patent ductus into the lungs instead of going from the aorta to the rest of the body. Therefore, if the doctors find bounding pulses, then look at the chest and see hyperactive beating of the heart, and note a widening pulse pressure, they will be quite sure the infant has PDA even though they can't hear it.

PDA may also be diagnosed with noninvasive radiographic procedures. X-rays may be used to determine if the heart is enlarged and if there is a notable increase in the blood flow to the lungs. If so, PDA may be present. The diagnosis may also be made with the use of an echocardiogram; this is a type of sonogram that looks at the structure and function of the heart and the patent ductus itself. This, along with Doppler flow studies, can measure the amount of blood going through the ductus to the aorta through the pulmonary artery, and set up a ratio relationship between the amount of blood going to the body and the amount of excess blood going to the lungs. This can all be done in color and can be recorded on tape for careful review. These recent technological advances in radiographic equipment and image processing give the baby's attending physician, along with the pediatric cardiologist, an excellent view of cardiac structures even in the small premature baby. They have virtually eliminated the need for invasive cardiac catheterization for diagnostic purposes.

Some preexisting prematurity-related complications can increase the likelihood of persistent PDA, and therefore babies with these complications are continuously monitored for signs of the open ductus. If, for example, the preemie has anemia (page 84), the heart will have to work much harder to get oxygenated blood cells to all the tissues of the body. This extra burden on the heart will often aggravate a PDA. Also, babies with respiratory distress syndrome (RDS, page 34) will have an open ductus that initially allows the blood to flow freely from left to right and right to left without causing any problems while they are being treated with oxygen or a respirator. But when the baby recovers from RDS the pulmonary pressure will drop as it should and the blood will begin to shunt from left to right, sending excessive amounts of blood to the lungs and causing further respiratory problems. The baby may need to go back on supplemental oxygen or the respirator, and his doctors will then look for evidence of PDA complication. If the PDA is not treated, the baby may eventually become oxygen or respirator dependent because every time he is taken off the respiratory aid, the respiratory problem will recur.

Treatment

There are three common courses of treatment for patent ductus arteriosus. The first and most desirable is most effective with the larger and more mature preemie. It entails improving oxygenation with an oxygen hood, or very often with CPAP or a respirator. This is done while limiting fluids, and/or drawing out excess fluids from the lungs, and being patient. Often with this medical therapy the ductus will dramatically decrease in size, thereby limiting the amount of blood being allowed to flow directly to the lungs. This is sometimes all that is needed to control the problem until the ductus closes completely on its own.

If this treatment is not effective, or if the blood flow to the lungs severely endangers the baby's state of health and therefore patience is not an option, medication may be used to treat PDA. There are a number of aspirinlike medications that tend to decrease the size of the open ductus. A drug called indomethacin (trade name Indocin) is commonly used. Given intravenously or through an NG tube, indomethacin provides rapid improvement (within twelve or twenty-four hours) in 50 to 70 percent of affected babies. However, this medication therapy has some negative side effects. It may also close other blood vessels in the body that need to remain open. Also, it may not be a safe drug for babies who have bleeding problems (such as intraventricular hemorrhage, page 99) because, as with any aspirinlike drug, it can promote further bleeding.

For those infants (usually the smaller, more immature and critically ill preemies) who cannot be treated successfully with the usual medical therapy or with medication, surgical ligation (closure) of the open ductus may be necessary. In this case, the baby will be given general anesthesia by an anesthesiologist who is specially trained to care for infants and children. Then, in the operating room, a surgeon who is specially trained in the diseases and treatment of the heart in young children (a pediatric cardiovascular or thoracic surgeon) will make an incision about 2 to 3 inches long between two ribs. He or she will then spread the rib cage wide open and move the lungs out of the way to gain full access to the blood vessels near the heart. (This operation does *not* in any way touch the heart muscle itself.) The surgeon will stitch through and around the ductus that connects the aorta to the pulmonary artery to tie it closed. He or she will then reposition the lungs and ribs, and close the incision. During the postoperative period the baby will be given pain relief medication, and a chest tube may be used to draw out any air or blood that may have accumulated in the chest cavity during surgery.

Medical therapy and medication are the preferred methods of treatment for PDA because any surgery, of course, puts stress on the body systems. But complications resulting from this operation are infrequent; and babies usually tolerate it quite well and respond with an immediate improvement in their health.

For some babies, time and patience are all that is needed to treat PDA. But for the majority of small, immature preemies, early medical intervention has generally been found to shorten the length of hospitalization, prevent chronic lung disease, limit the baby's time on supplemental oxygen and/or a respirator, and ultimately improve pulmonary outcome. Once the patent ductus arteriosus is tightly closed, it will not open again, and the infantile PDA will not predispose the child to any future heart problems.

RETINOPATHY OF PREMATURITY (ROP)

Retinopathy of prematurity, or ROP (once called retrolental fibroplasia, or RLF), is an eye disease affecting one third of all premature infants (half of those born weighing less than 2 pounds 4 ounces). This condition involves the blood vessels that spread like a spider's web over the surface of the retina to supply it with oxygen and nourishment. These blood vessels start at the optic nerve in the back of the eye and grow around in all directions toward the front of the eye. The immature, budding blood vessels are genetically programmed to grow from areas of high oxygen content (where they are) to areas of low oxygen content (where there are no blood vessels). While in utero, this program is easily followed, and in a full-term infant it will be complete at birth. However, after a premature birth, exposure to the oxygen in room air or to supplemental oxygen therapy confuses the genetic program. The budding blood vessels may grow in an errant and erratic manner, and bleed into the eye structure, causing the for-

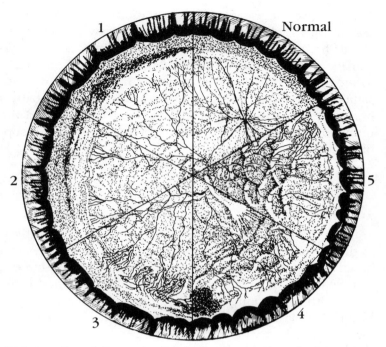

Retinopathy of Prematurity (This illustration depicts a normal eye, as well as five stages of progressive retinopathy of prematurity.)

mation of scar tissue. These scars may form behind the lens and block out light, and as they contract they may do damage to the retina. The resulting visual difficulties will be diagnosed as ROP.

It was once mistakenly believed that the administration of excessive amounts of oxygen was the only cause of eye problems in premature infants. Now it is known that it is not necessarily the administration of the oxygen that causes eye problems, but rather the fact of premature birth itself and immature retinal development. While a fetus is attached to the placenta, it exists on a very low oxygen level.

The increased level of oxygen in the bloodstream that occurs at birth, when the baby begins to draw oxygen from the air he now breathes, may be all that is necessary to do damage to retinal blood vessels that are not yet completely formed. With this discovery doctors have gained new insights into the need to monitor oxygen levels in the baby's body, and into the relationship between oxygen and the retinal development of all preemies regardless of their supplemental oxygen needs.

Diagnosis

An ophthalmologist (page 76) will examine your baby's eyes before he is discharged from the hospital. (If your baby is in the hospital for an extended period of time, his eyes will be examined at five or six weeks of age.) The routine eye examination is generally not an uncomfortable one for the baby, although, quite naturally, he will respond to the bright light and manipulation of the eye. It may, however, make you feel uncomfortable if you watch this exam, (even though it is a routine part of all normal eye examinations). The exam involves using eyedrops to dilate the pupil, and a lid retractor to hold the eye open. An instrument is then used to gently depress the sclera (white of the eye) to bring the entire retina completely into view through the pupil. This allows the ophthalmologist to see the complete circumference of the retina, to look for the orderly growth of the blood vessels over its surface.

Fortunately, in 90 percent of the cases, ROP will correct itself. In those few cases where this resolution does not occur on its own, treatment may be available to stop any damage to the visual system.

Treatment

If the ophthalmologist sees evidence of retinal detachment in a later stage of ROP, he or she may use a new and very effective procedure called cryotherapy to stop the abnormal growth of blood vessels that is pulling on the retina. After isolating the eye from the surrounding tissue (as described above), the doctor will use a tiny probe to freeze the abnormal growths, which by this time surround the entire eye. This is done under local anesthesia by touching the probe to the blood vessel through the outer surface of the eye; there is no cutting involved. Once the freezing procedure is completed, the abnormal blood vessels shrink and disappear, and new ones will grow normally. This procedure illustrates the kinds of major medical advances that have recently been made in premature baby care. If, just forty years ago, ROP progressed to the point where it began to detach the retina, doctors could do little more than stand by and watch the child's vision slowly deteriorate, sometimes to the point of blindness. At that time, the ophthalmologists could see that there was tissue growth behind the lens, but they didn't know what it was, or how it got there, or how to stop it from causing permanent damage.

In a small number of cases where the retina completely detaches even after freezing, or where advanced ROP was not detected because the baby was not taken for follow-up visits to the ophthalmologist, the child will undergo an operation to reattach the retina. This, of course, is a more complex procedure and points out why, since ROP can progress even after discharge from the hospital, it is very important to follow your doctor's advice about taking your baby for follow-up visits to the ophthalmologist.

By the time a preemie is "full-term," the retina and its blood vessels should be completely matured. If they have not grown together properly by this time, your baby may experience long-term nearsightedness (myopia), which can be corrected with glasses, or he may have permanent displacement or stretching of the retina, which will cause some vision distortion. (See "Dana's Story" on page 136.) If, however, the follow-up exam shows that the blood vessels have completely matured, as is most often the case, there is no further danger of regression, repetition, or development of prematurity-related eye problems.

BLOOD BANK INFORMATION

The hospital or local blood bank will supply the additional blood or blood components your premature baby may need during his stay in the hospital. This blood has been donated by people who have been screened for health complications that could affect the quality and/or use of their blood. It is also tested for the presence of infectious diseases such as hepatitis, syphilis, cytomegalovirus (CMV), and human immunodeficiency virus (HIV, which can cause AIDS). These precautions are taken to safeguard the quality of blood in the blood bank.

However, because there is a "window period" during which an infected unit of blood may test free of contamination, a very small amount (much less than even one percent) may unknowingly be made available to the general public. Because of this possibility, some parents will want to pick their own donor (called a directed or designated donor). If you want to do this, you should ask close friends and immediate family members to donate blood to the local blood bank immediately after the baby's birth. These people must meet the normal donor standards, which include:

• an acceptable hemoglobin level. (The baby's mother probably does not meet this criteria because of her own delivery-related blood loss.)

• a body weight over 110 pounds.
• no surgical procedures within the last six months.
• no history of IV drug use or homosexuality. (Even one exposure counts.)
• no medication unless approved by the blood bank.
• no evidence of CMV. (Nearly half of all adults carry this virus without symptoms or ill effects, but it could infect and cause complications in a premature baby.)

After the blood is drawn from the designated donor, it is sent to the lab for routine processing. It will take two or three days for it to be tested for contamination and labeled for group and type. When a donor with disease-free blood of a compatible type is found, one unit of whole blood will be drawn into a series of small bags. This blood will be good for thirty-five to forty-two days and will be enough for two to four transfusions. The same donor can contribute more blood, if needed, after an eight-week waiting period.

Using a designated donor sometimes makes parents feel more confident about the quality of the blood being given to their baby, but designated donors are not always a possible or desirable option. Because the processing of donated blood takes two to three days, designated donor blood cannot be used for medical procedures that must be done in the first day or two after birth. If, for example, the baby needs additional blood because he lost some in utero due to birth complications (such as placental abruption), or because he needs a transfusion to counter the effects of his mother's maternal antibodies, there may be no time to wait for a designated donor. Also, some very small, critically ill infants may need fresh blood, so designated donor blood that has been drawn and stored earlier is not usable. Designated donor blood may also be unusable if the baby needs blood components such as platelets, plasma, or fresh red cells. These cannot be extracted from the whole blood bags that were originally drawn and stored. If you know several days in advance that your baby will need a certain blood component, a designated donor can donate them at that time, but, again, because of the time factor, this can not be done in emergency situations.

If you want to use a designated donor, take great care in selecting that person. Out of desperation, some parents appeal at their place of employment, or through their church, or even in classified ads to whole populations of strangers. The window period that allows contaminated blood to pass undetected through the testing process can also affect the test results of designated donors. If someone close to you is able to donate blood that is compatible with your baby's blood type, this contribution will probably ease your mind. But if you can't locate a donor who is very well known to you, you should feel confident about using the blood from the local blood bank. As stated earlier, this blood is more thoroughly tested and therefore safer today than at any other time in history.

Chapter Four

. . . .

Very-Very Premature Babies*

25 to 29 Weeks Gestational Age

Babies who are born at 25 to 29 weeks gestational age (15 to 11 weeks early) are called very-very premature or very-very low-birth-weight babies.* Most often these babies weigh between 600 and 1600 grams (approximately 1 pound 5 ounces to 3 pounds 8½ ounces), and on the average they are 11 to 17 inches long. Their survival rate varies: Those born closer to 25 weeks and who weigh less than 2 pounds have a 50 to 70 percent chance of survival. Those born at 29 weeks have a 90 to 95 percent chance of survival.† These figures explain why such inten-

---

*All terms and medical procedures mentioned in this chapter have been explained in detail in other parts of the book, or are defined in the Glossary. Use the cross-references or the Index to find the pages that give more detailed information.

†This statistic excludes those babies born with the kinds of birth defects that are not directly related to prematurity. Defects such as chromosomal abnormalities, or severe heart or brain defects also affect the survival rates of full-term infants.

sive efforts are made to stop or prolong premature labor at a stage when every hour in utero increases the baby's chances of survival.

PHYSICAL APPEARANCE

The very-very premature baby looks like you would expect a fetus in utero to look at this same age. His head is disproportionately large in comparison to his total body size. His skin is wrinkled and has a red-purplish tinge. It also has a gelatinlike transparency that makes the surface arteries and veins clearly visible. You may notice bruises on the baby's skin. These can be caused by the slight pressure of the monitor leads against the skin or even by the touch of your finger. Without the layers of fat that full-term babies are born with, the very-very premature infant appears quite skinny and bony. He has soft lanugo hairs all over his body and his scalp hair is coarse. His eyeballs bulge out against eyelids that often don't have eyelashes. This baby's ears lie close against his head and have little or no cartilage, so if the ear flap is folded down it may stay down. He has just the beginning buds of soft finger- and toenails and has no creases on the soles of his feet.

Even at this earliest level of prematurity, the male and female sexual organs are clearly differentiated. However, the male's testes have not yet descended into the scrotum, and the female's clitoris protrudes out from the surrounding labia and her vaginal area is fully exposed because the outer folds of protective skin are not yet fully grown. Neither will have breast nipples or breast tissue under the skin, but there may be signs of the developing areola (the circle of dark skin around the nipple).

The very-very premature baby has negligible muscle tone. He does not lie in the expected fetal position, but rather with his arms and legs flat out at his sides. If you were to lift an arm or leg off the bed and then let it go, it would flop back down to the mattress. These babies will offer little resistance to forced movement of the limbs.

BODY TEMPERATURE CONTROL

Temperature control is a primary concern for very-very premature babies. They have virtually no fat tissue to help regulate their internal body temperature, and so these babies must always be artificially warmed on a radiant warmer or in an incubator. In addition, you may see the baby lying under heat shields. (They look like the sun reflectors people use to get a suntan.) These shields intensify the heat from the artificial heat source. The smallest of preemies may even be wrapped in cellophane to preserve whatever body heat they may generate. Usually these babies are also breathing through a tube that connects to a respirator, so their entire bodies (head and all!) can be wrapped up. If your baby gets the cellophane treatment, you'll probably feel better about this approach to temperature control if you view the plastic wrap as a see-through blanket rather than a sandwich covering.

RESPIRATORY CARE

It is possible that a very-very premature baby could have lungs that are developed enough to enable him to breathe without any respiratory assistance. However, this would certainly be an exception to the rule. Generally, the very-very premature infant needs some kind of respiratory equipment to help his lungs take in air and exhale carbon dioxide. Some may need only the supplemental oxygen supplied through an oxygen hood (page 34); others may need the more active help of CPAP (page 35); many will initially need the aid of a respirator (page 35). Whichever kind of respiratory support is used, these infants will have much more difficulty breathing than older preemies. As you watch them struggle for breath, you'll notice acute sucking in of the chest, flared nostrils, and grunting noises. For them, breathing is a very tiring activity.‡

Just when these babies are over the respiratory distress period (usually sometime in the first week of life), they will probably begin to have periodic breathing pauses (apnea, page 31). For you, the parents of the very-very premature baby, this is the beginning of the many good news/bad news days that lie ahead. The good news is that now the lungs are improving and the baby can breathe more easily with less supplemental oxygen; the bad news is that now the immaturity of the respiratory and neurological systems will periodically cause the baby to stop breathing. These apnea episodes will occur on and off for several weeks. It is scary to hear that your baby will occasionally stop breathing, but actually it is rarely a cause for serious concern. When the baby's breathing rate slows down below an acceptable level, the apnea monitor sounds its alarm. If the baby does not quickly resume breathing, the nurses will stimulate him to resume a normal breathing pattern. See page 31 for a more detailed discussion of apnea.

FEEDING METHODS

Very-very premature babies cannot suck, swallow, and breathe at the same time. Therefore, unlike full-term babies, they cannot immediately be breast- or bottle-fed. Al-

---

‡As explained in Chapter Two, sometimes a baby must be sedated or partially paralyzed while on intermittent ventilation to keep him from fighting against the inflow of air. In these cases the babies do not show signs of labored breathing.

most all of these babies will begin their nutritional intake with an intravenous glucose solution. Then, when their electrolytes (sodium, potassium, and calcium levels) are stable and they show a tolerance for the glucose solution (usually within three days), they are switched either to an IV solution of total parenteral nutrition (page 37), or to breast milk or formula feedings through an NG tube that is threaded through their nose or mouth down to their stomach (page 42). They will continue the NG tube feedings until they are approximately 34 weeks postconceptual age. At that time they will be introduced gradually to the bottle or breast.

If the very-very premature baby's mother wants to breast-feed, she should be sure to mention this to the doctors and nurses right after the baby's birth. They will instruct her how to express and store her milk while the baby is on IV solutions. (Also see Chapter Eight). This will keep up her milk supply so that when the baby is ready for oral feedings through the NG tube, she will be ready to provide the milk.

BEHAVIOR

Babies who are born 15 to 11 weeks early spend about 80 percent of their day sleeping. Although persistent prodding may cause them to open their eyes for a few seconds, they cannot see as you do. They see contrasts of light and dark and seem to be able to focus on black straight lines against a white background. Most often they can't stay awake long enough for any social interaction.

Studies have also found that these babies do not have fully developed olfactory or auditory functioning. Most often they do not react at all to pleasant or pungent smells, and although they could hear in utero sounds at about 17 weeks, now they may not startle at loud sudden noises.

Considering these facts, it's amazing but true that your very-very premature baby knows when you're with him.

These babies cannot cry to call for your attention or to express discomfort, but you can see evidence of excitement or distress by observing physical changes such as: a pale or blue skin color, a body posture that is excessively stiff or limp, an arching back, repeated yawning or hiccupping, flailing arms and legs, and/or a decrease or increase in heart or breathing rate. The "Parenting Tips" discussed later will tell you how to soothe your baby when you notice these reactions to environmental stimuli.

The very-very premature baby has limited muscle tone and does not move spontaneously very often. But just as you could feel his movements in utero, he will still occasionally bend and stretch his limbs, or clasp his fingers into a fist and then spread them wide open. He may even try to bring his hands close to his mouth to suck on his fingers.

Your tiny baby may not show much behavioral activity, but he is alive. His body systems are all working hard to help him adjust to life outside the uterus and to grow in size and strength. Just as he would have grown stronger one day at a time in the uterus if he had not been born early, so too he will grow now—slowly but surely, one day at a time.

TRANSFER INFORMATION

Babies born between the twenty-fifth and twenty-ninth week of gestation will usually need immediate intensive medical care to stabilize all vital signs and to provide respiratory assistance as needed. These babies almost always require the kind of equipment, personnel, and round-the-clock intensive care found in Level III and in some Level II facilities. If a very-very premature baby is born in a Level I or a Level II hospital without an in-house neonatologist, the baby will be transferred to a higher level medical center.

Very often, in fact, when a woman goes into labor at this stage of her pregnancy, she is sent to a Level II or III hospital for delivery. There she has the benefit of high-risk obstetric experts who may be able to prolong the pregnancy successfully. Then, when the baby is born, he will not have to be separated from his mother, or endure the trauma and delay of transport.

PARENTING TIPS

The extent of your immediate involvement in the care of your very-very premature baby depends on his state of medical stability. Check with the baby's doctors and nurses before you try any of the suggestions in this chapter. Although you probably will not be able to hold your child in your arms, once his vital signs are stabilized there are some things you usually are able to do to comfort and care for your baby.

Even the tiniest premature babies have distinct personalities as well as likes and dislikes. Through trial and error, you'll soon find out which of the following activities are comforting to your child, and which ones are distressing. He'll let you know by showing the signs of stress mentioned earlier. Very-very premature babies need lots of sleep, and because of their immature central nervous system, they are very easily overstimulated. You can reduce the risk of stressing your baby by trying only one activity at a time, and then waiting about three hours before you try another. If you talk to him *and* stroke his legs *and* tap on the glass of the incubator all at the same time, it will probably be too much for him to handle and he'll respond with distress signals. Always approach your baby slowly,

gently, quietly, and confidently, and then you can try the
following:

• Offer your baby physical contact by placing your finger
in his hand. Some very-very premature babies will have
developed their grasp reflex and will hold on to your finger.
• Rest your open hand over the baby's back and head.
He's not ready for a back rub yet, but just the feel of your
warm hand can be very comforting.
• If your baby is strong enough to suck, ask the doctor
if he can have a pacifier; the nursery may have special
preemie-size pacifiers or dummy nipples he can use. You
might also be able to calm your baby by letting him suck
on your pinky finger. If you want to try this, be sure your
hands are washed thoroughly and your nail is very short.
You can also position the baby's hands near his mouth so
that he can suck his own fingers if he wants to.
• Sometimes you'll see rolled-up towels at the baby's
sides and feet. These help him maintain his position and
provide a sense of comforting closeness. If the nurses are
very busy, they may not be able to keep the towels in place
all the time. You can do this for your baby. Don't put them
near his face, or squish them too tightly against him. Just
let them touch his skin slightly so he can feel them.
• Watch the nurses handle your baby. Watch how they
hold his arms and legs close to his body as they slowly
change his position. Watch how they maneuver around the
monitoring wires to bathe and diaper him. Watch closely
because very soon—when the baby is stable and you feel
confident—you yourself will be doing these things for him.
Also, as you get to know the nurses, you'll probably learn
a not-so-well-kept secret: Even when you're not yet allowed to hold the baby, "somebody" has to hold him while
the nurses change his bedding, and "somebody" has to
carry him to the scale for his daily weigh-in. If you happen

to be in the nursery at these times, that "somebody" could probably be you. Ask one of his nurses. It's worth a try.

If your baby doesn't want to be touched, and he doesn't want a pacifier, and he won't open his eyes to look at you, don't worry about it. Talk to him softly; he remembers your voice from his time in the uterus. But if even that seems to distress him, just let him rest. That's probably what he'd be doing if he were still being carried in the womb.

These ideas are specifically for parenting the very-very premature baby. In addition, be sure to read about the many other things described in Chapter Eight that you will be able to do for your baby as he grows.

Dana's Story

by Nancy Liljegren

My pregnancy was progressing normally. Because I was thirty-seven years old, I had an amniocentesis test at the appropriate time and found out that I was carrying a healthy little girl. My husband, Bruce, and I were delighted that the child was healthy and that we were going to have a daughter because we already had two sons, Erik (age eleven) and Keith (age eight).

One night, thirteen weeks before my due date, my labor contractions began as I was driving out to the airport to pick up relatives. When I got home and went to the bathroom I passed a lot of blood. I knew something was very wrong, so Bruce and I went right to the hospital. My obstetrician told me that the contractions could not be stopped. I vividly remember him saying it was unlikely that a baby born at 27 weeks gestation could survive. Nonetheless, he felt that a cesarean delivery might increase the baby's chances of surviving the trauma of birth, so he scheduled my delivery for eight o'clock that night. I didn't cry at the time, but I felt empty and desperate inside. I wanted so much to have this daughter and now I was being told she might die. One hour later, on May 24, 1983, Dana Lee was born weighing 2 pounds 4 ounces and measuring 14 inches long.

Dana had to be transferred to a hospital that had an intensive care nursery. Just before she left, her doctor suggested (actually, he insisted) that I see the baby. I was surprised to see a miniature, though complete, infant with rosy-yellowish skin. It seemed unbelievable to me that she was alive. Our visit lasted only a few minutes, then it was time for her to go. Bruce followed the transfer vehicle to the new hospital. There, he was told, she had about a 60 percent chance of survival. (At that point, 60 percent

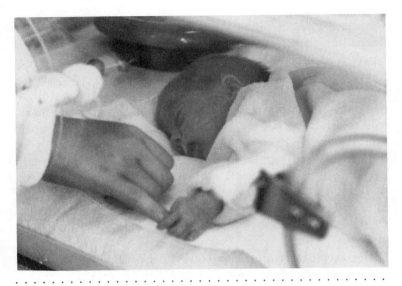

Dana at three weeks (The hand belongs to her eight-year-old brother, Keith.)

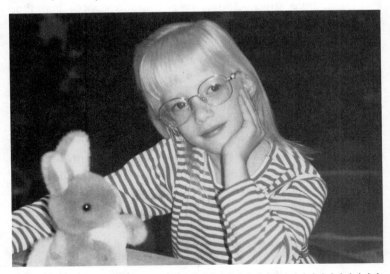

Dana at age six.

sounded wonderfully optimistic.) Then at about 2 A.M. I heard him in the hall outside my room. As he approached I prepared myself for the worst. My first words as he entered were "Is she dead?"

Bruce said, "No, but it's too early to tell how she might progress." He described the intensive care nursery, and he told me that the baby was stable for now. The doctors told him that the first twenty-four to forty-eight hours were very critical. I would not let myself believe that she really might live for very long. I was afraid to even hope that she'd still be living five days later when I'd be released from the hospital and able to see her. Even when the doctor encouraged us to name the baby, inside I kept feeling, "What's the point?!"

The day I was released from the hospital, Bruce and I went immediately to see Dana. All the way there I kept wondering what she'd look like. It was hard to imagine anything smaller than what I had seen when she was born, but since then she had lost weight and was now less than 2 pounds. I also worried about how I would feel when I finally saw my daughter—the little girl I had wanted so desperately but whom I was now afraid to even think about loving.

At first I was intimidated by the nursery. This was not a dimly lit, quiet place with soft lullabies gently putting little babies to sleep. It was bright, humming with activity, and it seemed very mechanical. Dana was sleeping and didn't seem to mind, but it took time and the help of understanding doctors and nurses before I could feel comfortable there. I was also bothered by the monitoring wires that were attached to Dana; they seemed so ominous and threatening. But as I grew more comfortable with the whole environment, the monitors actually gave me a sense of security. Eventually, it became the thought of taking Dana away from this protective environment that was frightening.

Three days later, just as I was beginning to hope that Dana might really live, she developed an infection. The neonatologist explained the causes and treatment and possible consequences. Although he tried his best to reassure us, this was still an emotional setback for me. Now, without being able to give up hope for Dana's survival, I had to accept how tentative her existence really was. Fortunately, Dana responded well to the treatment and recovered quickly. The fact that she had been able to recover from this problem gave me the strength I needed to handle each of the following setbacks as they came.

One of Dana's ongoing complications was an open blood vessel in her heart. (The doctor called this patent ductus arteriosus, or PDA for short.) She was given medication to help close it, but its administration had to be carefully monitored to be sure it wouldn't affect her respiration, which was just now holding its own. This, along with discussing her blood gas analysis and weight gain, comprised most of our daily conversations with the doctors.

Dana also had recurring spells of apnea. It was very frightening for me to leave the nursery knowing that she frequently stopped breathing, and worrying that one of these times the nurses wouldn't be able to revive her. I also wondered if these breathing pauses could cause brain damage, but her doctors assured me that the spells didn't last long enough for this to happen. Finally, after a few weeks, she stopped having this problem.

Six weeks after her birth, a pediatric ophthalmologist checked Dana's eyes. He found that both her eyes were affected by ROP (retinopathy of prematurity). He said that sometimes this disease is caused by the excessive amounts of supplemental oxygen some preemies need. Since Dana had received only a minimal amount of supplemental oxygen, in this case the problem was probably due to exposure to the normal atmospheric oxygen level. He said this commonly happens because the eyes of premature babies are just not ready for full oxygenation. Dana immediately had surgery (called cryosurgery) to freeze the abnormal blood vessels that were pulling on the retina of her right eye, the one that seemed to be most severely affected. A week later the same procedure was repeated on the left eye. The scariest part about this operation was the fact that Dana had to be paralyzed before the surgery could be performed. The neonatologist spent hours convincing Bruce and me that this was absolutely necessary. Although we finally agreed, I worried about the paralysis throughout the surgery and then again over the following twenty-four hours while we waited for her to get back to "normal."

Throughout Dana's stay in the nursery, Bruce and I were encouraged to make contact with her even while she was in the incubator. We were told it was good to talk to her and to touch her. Her brothers drew pictures that we taped on the incubator, and we placed a small music box near her. It seemed that she was becoming more of a "real" baby when we could finally dress her in preemie clothes. And then the biggest thrill came when she weighed 3 pounds 5 ounces, and we were able to remove her from the incubator, wrap her warmly, and hold her. We have wonderful photos of each of us, Keith and Erik too, holding her as we sat in a big rocking chair. The miracle of the moment shines through those pictures.

Finally on August 14, eighty-two days after her birth, we brought Dana home weighing 4 pounds 11 ounces. During Dana's hospitalization there had been so much to think about every day that it wasn't until we were home and settled into a daily routine that we began to consider any long-term developmental problems. During the first week we were home, and frequently thereafter, we took Dana to see the ophthalmologist who had performed the eye surgery. When she was about six months old, he suggested more eye surgery. We consulted with another doctor who advised us to wait, and he prescribed glasses for her to wear when she reached nine months of age. Dana continues to wear glasses. Sometimes she wears various kinds of patches over her right eye, or, she wears glasses that have a slightly opaque film over the right lens. This forces her to use the much weaker left eye. It's a battle to keep the glasses on her because she sees better with the right eye and she doesn't want the film covering it. However, her doctor feels we are making some progress in our efforts to strengthen the left eye.

Dana returned to the hospital's developmental center for periodic checkups. I distinctly remember the visit when she was seven months old. The neonatologist and the neurologist were concerned because Dana rarely smiled and her small and large motor skills were not age-appropriate. They recommended that we see a developmental specialist every two weeks. The therapist could monitor her progress and teach me how to help her develop large and small motor skills. After a while we began seeing the therapist every week, and we also began going to the Cerebral Palsy Center for weekly therapy sessions. It could not yet be determined if Dana had cerebral palsy, but her doctors and therapists felt that the early intervention program offered at the center would be helpful in fostering developmental skills. At this point, I was worried about Dana's future, but at the same time I knew I was doing everything possible to help her develop to her full potential. Today, I'm certain that our work with the therapists at such an early age was fundamental in helping Dana avoid larger problems. All children need lots of love and attention, but it seems that preemies need an extra dose to help them become the best they can be. The effort was exhausting at times, but it's good to look back now and know that we did all we could for our child.

Just before her first birthday, Dana seemed to "wake up."

She became more involved with people and things, and she began to fall within the realm of "normal" development. For the next two years we continued intensive physical therapy sessions, but by the end of her first year we were feeling very lucky. Dana was keeping up with age-related developments in major areas, and cerebral palsy seemed a less likely possibility. She was able to sit and stand; she was learning to walk and talk, and she was happy.

When Dana was three years old she stopped all physical therapy sessions and we enrolled her in a local nursery school program for three- and four-year-olds five mornings a week. She also began a gymnastics class which helped her continue to develop her large motor skills. She had graduated to being a regular kid on the block—with glasses.

Dana did not begin public school kindergarten when she was five years old. The developmental group at the hospital did a major evaluation of her when she turned five. They found her verbal and number-concept skills to be advanced for her age, but because of her underdeveloped small motor skills and her vision problems (which caused her to shy away from coloring and drawing letters), they suggested that we wait one more year before beginning kindergarten. This year she went to a private transitional kindergarten where she has blossomed to the point where she is ready for public school next fall.

Dana is now six years old and weighs forty-three pounds. Her vision remains her basic handicap, but we are so grateful she can at least see. Without the cryosurgery, she might have been blind. Sometimes I look at her in her "dress-up" clothes having a tea party with her friend, or watch her running across the yard, and I think how wonderful it is to have such a loving, healthy, happy child. And I marvel that she started life so early and so little.

Dana's birth was traumatic, but looking back on it, I realize that her problems were relatively few and her doctors, nurses, therapists, and everyone else involved in her care were wonderful. I regret that Dana was born prematurely because her eyes would be better if she'd remained in utero longer. However, given the circumstances, Dana and all of us who love her are extremely fortunate that she was born at a time when medical science could give her life.

Kevin's Story

by Rosalind McGrady

I was twenty-five years old and unmarried when I became pregnant. The baby's father was unable to accept my pregnancy and did not want a baby at that time. But I wanted this baby so I decided to go it alone. I had a normal pregnancy, and I never once thought about delivering early. I would sometimes think (like all pregnant women) about the possibility of having a child who was born without a limb, or one who was born deaf, or blind, or even stillborn, but I never once thought about one who would come early.

I went into labor in the morning on July 27, 1984; this was 14 weeks before my due date. By the time I got to the doctor's office it was too late for him to do anything except call for an ambulance. Kevin was born that same morning at 9:33 A.M. at a nearby hospital. He weighed 1 pound 11 ounces and was 13 inches long.

I was lying on the delivery table watching as they inserted an IV into my baby and attached monitoring wires, and gave him forced supplemental oxygen to help him breathe. Even though I'm a nurse, and I knew what was going on, I've never been so scared in my life. The only thing that kept me from panicking was watching his little arms and legs as they were kicking wildly in the air. From the moment I saw that, I knew he wasn't going to die. I can't explain why, but I never once considered death as a possibility. I believe that my faith in God has gotten me through every terrifying moment.

Kevin was breathing a little on his own, but the doctors put him on a respirator to help him take in adequate amounts of oxygen, and they made arrangements to transfer him to another hospital where there was an intensive care nursery. The fact that Kevin had to be taken away from me was probably the most awful experience of all. I

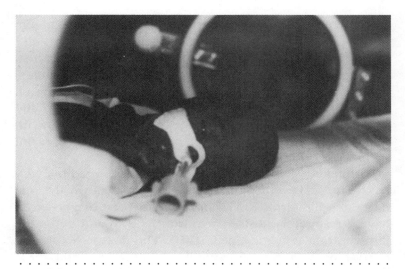

Kevin shortly after birth.

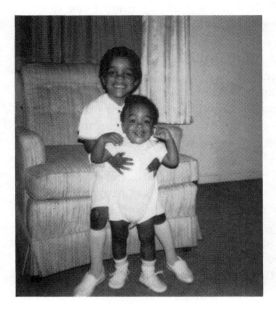

*Kevin at age five
with his younger
brother, Robert,
fourteen months
(He was also a
preemie!)*

can still remember when a nurse and a doctor wheeled him into my room. I looked at him, and through my tears all I could say was "He's so tiny." He was still kicking with all his might as I reached out to touch him, and he touched me. It was a wonderful feeling, but then it was time for him to go. There's nothing worse than sending your own child off to a place you know nothing about. I couldn't go with him, and I didn't know how long he'd have to stay. But then he was gone, and I was alone.

Fortunately, I was well enough to be discharged the very next day, so I went right to the new hospital. In the one day since his birth, Kevin already had been diagnosed as having respiratory distress syndrome (RDS) and a grade 4 intraventricular hemorrhage (IVH). The doctors explained everything to me very carefully. I knew all about these things because of my medical background, but at the time I was so scared, I needed them to tell me everything very slowly and in great detail.

Kevin was so small and so sick that one of the doctors asked me to think very carefully if I really wanted this child. He said that Kevin's care would be very extensive, and after all that, he might not live. I remember looking at that doctor with such anger and hurt. How could he even think that I wouldn't want him to do everything possible to keep my baby alive? I wanted Kevin to live more than anything else in the world, and I wouldn't "think carefully" about any other possibility. I knew in my heart that Kevin was not going to die.

This doctor was right about one thing: Kevin was in the hospital for a very long time and he had many setbacks. It seemed like every time he'd just recover from one problem, he'd develop another. Two weeks after his birth, Kevin developed something called necrotizing enterocolitis (NEC). Because of this, he had to have surgery to repair a perforated bowel. I still can't describe the fear I felt at just the thought of such a tiny baby having to have surgery. But even still, I knew he'd pull through—and he did.

A few weeks later, Kevin was back in the operating room. He had run out of veins to use for IV insertion sites, so the doctors put in a broviac catheter. This way he could get his fluids and nourishment through a tube that was inserted into a large vein in his neck and that came out through his chest. Once this was in place, Kevin did seem to start getting better, and he also began putting on some weight (although his weight gain was always an up-and-down battle).

One month later the doctors told me that they felt Kevin's irregular breathing pattern and heart rate were caused by a condition called patent ductus arteriosus (PDA). To correct this, he would need another operation that would regulate the flow of the blood from his heart to his lungs. ("Will it ever end?" I'd ask myself over and over.) Kevin had to be transferred to a big city hospital for the surgery. Again, I had to stand by and watch my child be taken away from me. I stood there wishing I could run right behind that ambulance rather than lose sight of him, but then he was gone. Early the next morning, I went to the hospital where the surgery was to be performed. I was upset about my baby having to have another operation, but when I got there I became furious. Kevin had already gone down to surgery and no one had called to tell me. The whole place was cruel and cold. There was a big wide-open room with all these babies hooked up to respirators and IVs. It seemed so impersonal and so different from the hospital he had come from. I just wanted to take my baby out of there as soon as possible. I stayed with him all night; then, the very next day, we went back to the other hospital. For the next few days Kevin had a tube coming out of his chest that helped his lungs to drain, and he was uncomfortable because the surgeon had to break a rib to get at his heart. But again, Kevin made it through like I knew he would.

The following month an ophthalmologist told me that my baby needed eye surgery. The blood vessels in Kevin's left eye were growing abnormally, and if left untreated he could lose sight in that eye. So Kevin then had cryosurgery, which freezes the abnormal blood vessels so they can't do further damage. This eye condition is called retinopathy of prematurity (ROP), and I've heard since that it's pretty common in preemies.

Just when it looked like Kevin was finally over the worst, he got an infection. Although he responded well to the antibiotics, he was put in isolation so that none of the other babies would catch it from him. It made me feel like an outsider. Kevin was put in a dark and quiet back room with only two or three other infected babies around. I was surprised that he adjusted so well because he had been used to the noise and lights of the intensive care nursery. But by now, I guess my baby could adjust to anything.

While all this was going on, I had a lot of adjusting to do myself. For the first three months I couldn't even hold my baby. After his operations, when he looked so frail and needy, I couldn't cradle him in my arms and press my cheek against his forehead and comfort him. All I could do was touch him through the porthole of the incubator. I would hold his little head in my hand because I couldn't hug him close to my heart. Sometimes I'd beg the nurses to let me hold him while they weighed him and changed his bed. Although he was still attached to a respirator, and I was very nervous, I'll never forget the time the nurse gave in and gently placed him in my arms. It was like holding just a blanket (he only weighed two-and-a-half pounds), but it was the first time he was all mine.

Being a single parent was especially difficult at this time. I wanted to be strong for my baby, but some days it seemed so endless, so tiring. Fortunately for me, the nurses in ICN were wonderful. They became a part of my family; they gave me hope, and strength, and even peace of mind. Kevin had a specially assigned nurse during each shift. I always knew who was taking care of him, and I trusted each one. I think they all came to love Kevin almost as much as I did. I also had the support and help of my mother. (She's the greatest!) I don't know how I would have made it through this time without her. I also found that the hospital social worker was very caring and had a lot of information that was very helpful to me. I had so much on my mind that I didn't think or care about money, but she did. She helped me organize my insurance forms and find other sources of financial aid. (I had no idea that the hospital stay would cost approximately $125,000, and the doctor bills would be about $30,000). Even after discharge she referred me to social services that I wouldn't have known about on my own. It was very nice having someone look after these things when I was too emotionally tired to do it for myself.

Throughout the seventeen weeks of Kevin's hospital stay, I did whatever I could to let him know I was there and that I loved him. I visited every day (sometimes three times a day), and I always talked to him and touched him. I would gently rub his dry skin with lotion; I really believe that this touching helped his recovery. I think there are factors in touching that make people heal better, and, of course, there's nothing better than a mother's touch. As little as Kevin was, he always could sense when I was there. The nurses even said that he would act up when I left—his heart rate would go down or his breathing would become irregular. Although Kevin didn't interact with me, it made me feel good to know he missed me.

It's hard to go to the hospital every single day and sit and sit and sit. One day a doctor looked at me sitting next to the incubator as I did every day, and he said, "Why don't you go back to work?" I guess he knew I needed something else to occupy my mind for at least a part of each day. So I took his advice and went back to nursing. I still spent time with Kevin every day, but working helped ease some of the tension.

Finally, when Kevin was 4 months 1 week old, and weighed 4 pounds 9 ounces, I talked the doctors into letting me take him home. I think they finally gave in because I'm a nurse and convinced them I could give him the care he needed. Actually, Kevin was doing very well by then. Although he had been on a respirator for ten weeks, and then on CPAP for ten days, he wasn't oxygen-dependent now, and so he didn't need any home-care equipment.

Once we were at home, I was a little nervous about being alone with him, but I knew I could do it. My mother was still helping me, and there was a visiting nurse who came once in a while to make sure we were okay. After everything Kevin had been through, I knew he'd be fine now. I spent the next six months at home with Kevin, but then I had to go back to work because my leave was over. I hated leaving him, but being a single parent I had to support myself and Kevin. I know that when he grows up, he'll understand and love me just the same.

We went back to the hospital regularly for extensive follow-up care. Kevin had checkups with the developmentalist, neurologist, physical therapist, ophthalmologist, neonatologist, and pediatrician. We also started an early intervention program that was offered at a local state college. All of this required a lot of time and running around, but I'm very glad that I never refused any of this help. I always thought that Kevin was progressing well, but when a child has had extensive brain hemorrhage, his long-term prognosis is not usually good, so I wanted him to have every advantage and opportunity possible. Today, I know that I did all I could to help him overcome his developmental delays. When I look at him now, I can't help but smile.

Now, Kevin is five and a half years old. He is thirty-eight inches tall and weighs thirty-two pounds. His only long-term health complication is mild right-sided cerebral palsy that is a result of the brain hemorrhage. For such an extensive bleed, he is doing remarkably well (certainly better than I was told he would do). He's able to run; he talks fluently; he's very intelligent, and to look at him you wouldn't think anything at all was wrong with him (at least not until you picked up his shirt and saw all his scars). He's been back in the hospital only twice in these five years. Once was for an intestinal virus, and then again for more surgery. There was evidence of increased swelling of his head and pressure on his brain from his hemorrhage. So he had a shunt put in for drainage. This was very hard for me to deal with because after three and a half years I thought Kevin was past the point where he could suffer any more from his hemorrhage. Despite my worries, the surgery went well and now he's doing fine again. Kevin still goes to the early intervention program at the hospital, and to the developmental clinic. Although we still see the ophthalmologist occasionally, Kevin's eyes have completely recovered from ROP. He also goes to a preschool for handicapped children and is progressing very well.

Kevin is the joy of my life. I can't imagine living without him. As I look at the tiny footprint they took at his birth, it amazes me to think he could have been that small. But I know he was, and I know I'll never forget those weeks that he lived in the hospital. It was the most painful and frightening time of my life.

Since Kevin's birth I have married a wonderful man who loves Kevin just as much as I do. Since we didn't want Kevin to be an only child, I again became pregnant. Again, 13 weeks early I went into labor. I could not believe the nightmare was starting all over again. This time my obstetrician was able to hold off my delivery for one extra week, and I'm amazed at the difference that one week made. My second preemie was born weighing a buxom 2 pounds 6 ounces. He needed no major surgery at all, just a cut-down for his IV and then some extra time to grow strong. My past experiences with Kevin prepared me for this second trip through ICN parenting, but again it was a difficult way to start out with a new baby.

Having been through "preemie parenting" twice, I have two pieces of advice I would like to offer other parents who are now in that situation. The first is: Don't be afraid to ask questions; knowledge is strength. The more you know, the more comfortable you'll feel about what's going on. You might wonder if you'll be bothering the nurses or the doctors with your questions, but ask anyway. It's your child, and no one loves him and cares for him like you do. My second piece of advice is: Don't ever give up hope. Love your baby; let him know you're there. You'll be amazed how much he'll fight to stay alive. Then, five years from now, like me, you'll have a wonderful, into-everything, beautiful child.

Chapter Five

Very Premature Babies*
30 to 34 Weeks Gestational Age

Babies who are born at 30 to 34 weeks gestational age (10 to 6 weeks early) are called very premature.* Most often these babies weigh between 1000 and 2500 grams (about 2 pounds 3 ounces to 5 pounds 8 ounces), and on the average they are 14 to 18½ inches long. Their survival rate is 90 to 95 percent.†

*All terms and medical procedures mentioned in this chapter have been explained in detail in other parts of the book, or are defined in the Glossary. Use the cross-references or the Index to find the pages that give more detailed information.
†This statistic excludes those babies born with the kinds of birth defects that are not directly related to prematurity. Defects such as chromosomal abnormalities, or severe heart or brain defects also affect the survival rates of full-term infants.

PHYSICAL APPEARANCE

The further from term a baby is born, the more immature his physical development will be. The very premature child, therefore, more closely resembles the younger, very-very premature baby than the older, moderately premature or full-term baby. The head of the very premature baby is proportionately much larger than his body. He has very thin skin, which appears translucent and which may still have a red-purplish tinge (pigmentation usually develops during the thirty-fourth week of gestation). He will appear "skinny" because he has not yet developed insulating layers of body fat, and he will also still have soft lanugo hairs on his body (especially on his back). The ears of a very premature baby will not spring back if folded down because they don't have enough firm cartilage, and the soles of his feet don't have as many creases as those of full-term babies.

Both the male and female very premature baby will have clearly differentiated sexual organs. However, the male's testes will not yet have descended into the scrotum, and the scrotum itself will be much smoother in appearance than it is in an older baby. The female preemie will have an exposed clitoris because the outer folds of protective skin will not yet have grown over her vaginal area. Neither will have breast nipples nor breast tissue under the skin, but there may be signs of the developing areola (the dark circle of skin around the nipple).

The muscle tone of a very premature baby is different from that of an older baby. Because he has very little muscle tone, he does not pull his arms and legs in close to his body in the common fetal position. Rather, he will lie with his arms and legs flat out at his sides like a frog. This lack of muscle tone allows the heel of his foot to be pulled up past his ears. As he grows, he will develop flexion that will resist this kind of movement.

The very premature baby has a lot of growing to do before his physical appearance can be compared to that of a full-term baby. Don't let this bother you; your baby is not yet full-term. He looks exactly as he should for his gestational age, and that makes him beautiful.

BODY TEMPERATURE CONTROL

Very premature babies have not yet developed the insulating layers of tissues and fat that will allow them to self-regulate their body temperature. These babies will always be warmed artificially on a radiant warming table or in an incubator. Their body temperature and their surrounding air temperature are constantly monitored to assure proper heat control. Because of their inability to self-regulate body temperature, a preemie will not be moved to an open-air cradle or bassinet until he is at least thirty-three to thirty-four weeks old, or four pounds.

RESPIRATORY CARE

Very premature babies are born with fully developed lungs. A few are able to breathe without any respiratory assistance, but most often the lungs are not mature enough to work effectively on their own. The degree of respiratory distress these babies will experience cannot, however, be predicted with any certainty. Some will need only supplemental oxygen; many will require CPAP assistance; still others will need complete ventilation from a respirator. The respiratory capabilities of a very premature baby are unique to each child. Therefore, your baby's doctors and nurses will carefully and constantly observe and monitor the baby's breathing patterns to determine the best way to maintain respiratory stability.

Even healthy, very premature babies have a higher-than-normal heart rate, a lower blood pressure, and occasional breathing pauses (apnea). If any of these conditions should deviate from their expected course, the nurses and doctors will be immediately alerted by the alarms of the monitors that are always attached to the baby.

FEEDING METHODS

Like all other preemies, the very premature baby will not be fed orally until the respiratory system is stabilized. While the doctors evaluate the baby's vital signs, as well as his digestive capabilities, his first "meal" will probably be glucose fluids or total parenteral nutrition (TPN). These are given through an IV or catheter line. They supply the baby with necessary nutrients and calories without challenging his digestive system.

Even when the respiratory system is stabilized, most likely the very premature baby will not be ready for nipple feedings. Although these babies have a well-developed rooting reflex that causes them to turn their head to look for food when they are touched on the mouth, they cannot yet coordinate the sucking, swallowing, and breathing sequence required for bottle- or breast-feedings. So when they are ready for oral feedings, most will begin with a naso-gastric tube. This NG tube (page 44) is threaded through the infant's nostrils or mouth down to the stomach. Then the baby is fed formula or breast milk from a small vial attached to the other end of the tube. Whether the baby is on an intermittent schedule of feedings every two to three hours, or is receiving round-the-clock nourishment from a continuous drip, very often the baby will be given a pacifier to suck during his feedings. This lets him practice his sucking, swallowing, and breathing coordination, and it is also believed to aid in the digestive and growth process.

Let the attending physician know if the baby's mother intends to breast-feed the very premature baby. While the baby is on IV fluids, she can express milk and freeze it. Then, when the baby advances to an NG tube, the breast milk can be used for these feedings. And finally, when the baby is approximately 34 weeks postconceptual age and ready for breast-feeding, his mother will have an ample supply of milk and will be able to meet his nutritional needs.

BEHAVIOR

Babies who are born 10 to 6 weeks early have an under-developed central nervous system. This is why, although they move more frequently than the younger, very-very premature babies, most of their movements and activities are halting, jerky, and unpurposeful. The very premature baby can grasp hold of your finger and can turn his head from side to side. But his neck muscles are too weak to hold his head up when he is pulled to a sitting position.

Some of these babies are still easily stressed by the stimulation of handling, talking, feeding, touch, or "play." A few are able to cry to express their discomfort, but most will show distress through changes in body signs, such as a blue or pale skin color, excessively stiff or lax muscle tone, an arching back, or changes in heart or breathing rate.

Very premature babies can stay awake for short periods of time that may begin as one- or two-minute excursions and grow to ten minutes or more. When awake they will open their eyes wide and will appear alert and watchful. These babies can see items within eight to ten inches of their face, and may fixate on one object for a while. They will turn away from a bright light and will seem more alert when their eyes are shielded from direct overhead lighting.

TRANSFER INFORMATION

It is difficult to say what level of hospital care will be necessary for a very premature baby. A very few may be born in good health without any special medical needs and therefore could be cared for by a pediatrician in a Level I facility. However, because the very premature baby is at risk for developing RDS and/or infections, even seemingly healthy babies are most often sent either to a Level II hospital with an in-house neonatologist or to a Level III intensive care nursery. The attending pediatrician will decide when and where to send a baby based on his needs and the location of nearby Level II and Level III facilities. Babies who are born in a Level I hospital and who show any instability in their vital signs will be immediately transferred to a higher-level care center.

PARENTING TIPS

Most very premature babies begin their interaction with their parents while confined to the warming table or incubator. If, at first, you cannot hold your baby, don't shy away from parenting him. There are still many things you can do to get to know your baby, to soothe and comfort him, and to stay actively involved in his care.

Your touch, your voice, and your face are all that you need to interact with your baby. To begin, you must first keep in mind that the awake period of a very premature baby is quite short. Ask the nurses if your baby has any predictable periods of wakefulness and, if so, try to schedule your visits at those times. If his sleep schedule is still unpredictable, your chances to interact will be hit-and-miss for a while. If he is sleeping when you visit, let him rest; continuous jostling of a preemie can hinder his efforts to sleep and grow. If he is awake when you visit, take advantage of the opportunity, but start slowly and stay alert for the signs of overstimulation mentioned earlier.

The best time to "play" with your baby is when he is rested and calm. To avoid tiring him, start with just one form of stimulus at a time. Without talking or making him focus on your face, touch him. Let him grab hold of your finger, or softly stroke, rub, and feel his arms, legs, and body. Some professionals call this "infant massage" (see the details in Chapter Eight), but actually it falls far short of the muscle kneading or pounding commonly associated with "massage." Simply, the feel of your gentle touch can be very comforting to your very premature baby.

At another time, offer your face eight to ten inches from your baby's. Without talking or touching, try to get his attention and let him focus on you. Then, slowly move your head from side to side and watch to see if he follows you with his eyes. Thirty seconds of this exercise will help your baby develop his visual-coordination skills and will provide both of you with some "play" time.

Very premature babies have been known to turn to the sound of their parents' voice. Without touching or striving for eye contact, talk softly to your baby. It doesn't matter what you say; it's the sound and the soft tone of your voice that will stimulate and comfort him. You may even want to ask the attending physician if you can leave a small tape player in the baby's bed so that when you're not there, the nurses can play a tape of your voice.

As your baby grows and his central nervous system matures, you can begin to combine these activities. You can, for example, talk while you stroke his body, or sing and touch him while you establish eye contact. Your baby's response will let you know what he likes and how much is too much.

Eventually, you will be able to do these things as you hold your baby in your arms. Although a very premature baby may cry, startle, and flail his arms when your first pick him up, once he is swaddled securely in blankets, hears the sound of your voice, and feels the warmth of your body, he will usually relax and enjoy the physical contact. But remember: All babies react differently to social interaction, and some react differently from one moment to the next. If your baby does not want to be held, or talked to, or touched, and won't look at your face, don't despair. This is not at all uncommon. Sometimes, the very premature baby just wants to be left alone. This may be his way of getting the rest he needs to grow strong enough to go home, where the two of you will have lots of time together to touch, to talk, and to love each other. If your baby becomes distressed by your attention, leave him alone for a while and try again later.

These parenting tips are specific to the very premature baby. Be sure also to read about the many things you can do for a preemie that are detailed in Chapter Eight.

Kathleen's Story

by Bergman Li

I was not prepared for the premature birth of my daughter. I already had a two-and-a-half-year-old son who was delivered at term, and my checkups during this pregnancy didn't show anything wrong. When I started having labor contractions, I didn't think I was really going to have my baby then—I was still eight weeks away from my due date.

At the hospital my obstetrician said that he wanted to stop the contractions because the baby was not yet fully developed and shouldn't be born yet. He hoped to put off my delivery for at least another four weeks. So, for the next two days I lay on my left side and received medicine through an IV to calm the contractions. But on Saturday morning, the doctor said I was starting to dilate and so he wanted me to go to another hospital. He said there I could get a different kind of medicine that might stop my labor, and if that didn't work, at least my baby would be born in a place where he could get the best kind of intensive care.

Once I was admitted to the new hospital, a resident gave me shots of medicine every hour. He too hoped this would stop my labor, but my baby had plans of her own. After getting these shots for seven hours, the contractions became very hard and quick. Without much warning, at 11 P.M. on May 5, 1984, Kathleen was born right in the labor room with only a nurse there to help me. The nurse was very nervous and she was yelling for help. A resident came running into the room. He wrapped the baby in a blanket, cut the cord, and ran back out with my child in his arms. I didn't feel much like a new mother. Everything happened so fast and then my daughter was gone.

The next morning I learned that Kathleen weighed 4 pounds 6 ounces and that she was in the intensive care nursery because she had stopped breathing shortly after

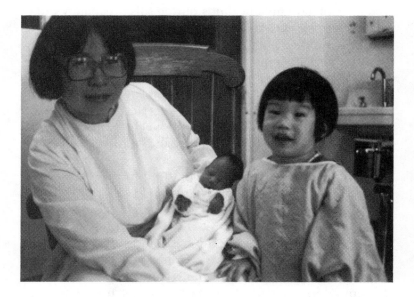

Kathleen at two weeks with her mom and brother, Jonathan, two and a half years

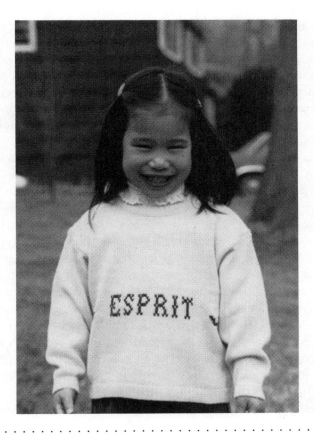

Kathleen at age five

she was born. She stayed there for three weeks because she kept having those breathing pauses and also because she had to gain weight before she could come home.

I was glad I was in the same hospital with her so that I could see her every day. At first it was hard to look at her because she was so tiny and had the wires attached to her. But then it was so hard to leave her when I was discharged from the hospital. Because I had my other child at home, it was difficult to spend as much time at the hospital with Kathleen as I would have liked, but I did manage to see her every day, even if it was only to whisper hello, and talk to the doctors about her progress. My husband also tried to see her on his lunch hour, and on the weekends we brought her brother, Jonathan. He was always thrilled to touch and hold his baby sister.

Finally, when Kathleen's weight was close to five pounds, she was ready to come home. (I don't know the exact weight because the doctor told it to me in grams.) I was so happy to have her at home with her family, but I was very worried that she would stop breathing again. The doctor told me that he did not think she would do that anymore, but if I wanted, I could tilt her mattress to keep her head higher than her feet. He said it might help her to breathe more easily and would stop the fluid or formula from backing up into her throat. Although I was very tired, I couldn't sleep well for the first few weeks she was home. Because I was worried that she'd stop breathing and I wouldn't know it, I kept getting up at night to check on her. I'd stand next to her crib, and rest my hand on her body to feel her breathing. Every breath was reassuring.

When Kathleen was discharged from the hospital the neonatologist told me to bring her back so the neurologist could do an ultrasound scan on her brain. We went back twice for these tests and a few more times for visits with the neurologist. I never got any reports or results back to let me know how Kathleen was developing, so we stopped going. When I think about it now, I realize I should have asked more questions and insisted on more answers. Fortunately, Kathleen has developed just as she should, and she doesn't have any learning problems. (When she was younger, she was shy and very attached to me, but I don't think that had anything to do with being premature.)

Once we were over the worry about the breathing pauses, I would not let myself think of anything negative. In fact, I have always tried to raise my daughter like a normal child. I do not feel I should do anything differently with her than I would do for my older son. Kathleen is now five years old; she weighs thirty-nine pounds, is forty-one inches tall, and her health is very good. She apparently has experienced no negative effects from being born eight weeks early. She goes to a regular nursery school five mornings a week where she is very outgoing and has lots of friends. She will begin kindergarten in September. Kathleen seems to be very bright and to have a special interest in music. She's been taking piano lessons since she was three years old. Now she can play many songs, and she has developed quite a musical ear. If she listens to a song a few times, she can then play it on the piano herself.

My family is Chinese. They have told me that children who are born at 32 weeks will be very smart. I don't think that's a scientific fact, but I do know that our Kathleen is a very smart, happy, and maybe even a musically gifted little girl.

David's Story

by Bonnie Dzendzel‡

George and I had been married for nine years when I became pregnant with our first child. I had an easy pregnancy. Except for the fact that I was widening around the middle, I was happy, healthy, and I felt fine. I had no morning sickness, no special cravings, and nothing out of the ordinary occurred. Despite this, the possibility of having a preemie occasionally crossed my mind because my mom's three children were all born prematurely. The first was a boy who was born 3 weeks early and weighed 5 pounds 14 ounces. The second was me. I was born 4 weeks early and weighed 5 pounds. The third was my sister who was born 5 weeks early and weighed 4 pounds 14 ounces. Fortunately, none of us suffered any complications. So, on December 23, 1984, when my water broke at five-thirty in the morning, although I was surprised, I wasn't at all worried. I know now that I was naive.

We met my obstetrician at our local hospital two hours later, and he confirmed that I was in labor. He told us that because our baby was going to be born early, he might suffer some respiratory distress. My husband and I said we understood, but at the time we really didn't know the full extent of what that could mean to our baby. My labor was easy; I still felt fine and was in a good mood. At about 11 A.M., I told the nurse I had this irresistible urge to push. She called in the doctor; he examined me and said, "Go ahead, push." So at 11:54 David was born weighing 4 pounds 10 ounces. He was 17½ inches long, and he had Apgar scores of 10, 10, and 9. David was absolutely fine.

‡Although this story is told by Bonnie Dzendzel in the first person, all of the information was gathered in a collaborative effort with her husband, George.

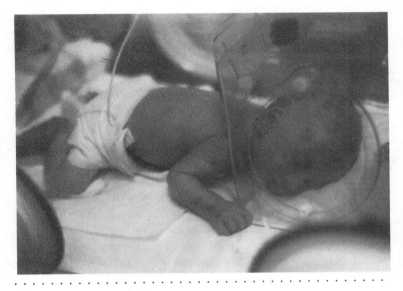

David at seven weeks

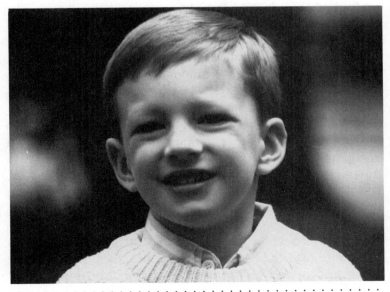

David at age four and a half

At four o'clock that afternoon I was on the phone announcing our good news to a friend when I heard an emergency page come over the PA system. Our pediatrician was being called to the nursery, and it occurred to me that something might be wrong with David. It was only a few minutes later when the pediatrician walked into my room and sat at the foot of my bed. Now I knew something was wrong. He told George and me that David had stopped breathing, that he had been resuscitated, and that he was being transferred to a different hospital. I could see George was upset so I tried to assure him by saying, "Don't worry. David will be fine." Then the doctor leaned forward, and in a strong yet concerned voice he slowly and deliberately said, "David is not fine. He has suffered respiratory distress and needs special medical attention." I'll never forget the sound of those words; they almost knocked me over. I kept hearing them over and over until I looked up and saw that David had been brought to my room in his incubator. The neonatologist who was taking charge of David during his transfer asked us if we wanted to hold David before he left. But we were too afraid; we both believed that if we took him out of his sterile environment, he would surely die.

David's move to the intensive care nursery left me feeling numb. I hadn't even planned to have a child at this time; now, before I had a chance to get to know him, he was moving away from me. I remember thinking that if David was going to die, it would be best if it happened now— now before I learned to love him. Once he was in the ICN, it was still difficult for me to feel close to him. Although we knew David was our son, it took a long time to really, deep down, believe that. He was in this isolated plastic box, with wires attached to his chest, with intravenous tubes going into his head and navel, and tubes from the respirator going into his nose. There were doctors and nurses, and respiratory and X-ray technicians constantly around him. His daily routine did not involve the usual changing diapers, feeding, and playing. It involved a constant poking and piercing of his body to obtain blood samples and gases. Eventually a central line catheter even had to be put in his arm because there were no more available veins. He had chest physiotherapy around the clock to help him breathe. X-rays were taken whenever a complication was suspected. Ultrasounds were taken to check for brain bleeds, and he even had a spinal tap at one point when an infection was suspected.

While all this went on, George and I sat next to his incubator feeling like outsiders. David's time in the intensive care nursery was the hardest time we have ever had to endure. For the first two weeks we couldn't even hold him. All we could do was put our arm through the porthole in his incubator and stroke David's head or arm—hardly the stuff that real parenting is made of, but it was all we could do to try to comfort him and let him know we were there for him. Trying to live day by day was very hard because we never knew what to expect. One day David would be doing well, and we'd hear only positive things. The next day, we'd hear that he was developing something that had to be carefully watched to see what procedures would be taken next. So many times I would come home and cry because I was casually told something that probably sounded innocent enough to the nurse or the doctor, but to me it was serious. I remember the day a nurse remarked, "David should be off the feeding solution by now. He can't stay on this much longer." What did that mean? What would happen if he didn't get off it; would he die? Another day, a neonatal fellow said that she'd noticed David hadn't been moving around much in his incubator. "He seems to just lie there," she said. "Maybe it's because he stopped breathing the day he was born." What were they telling me now? I felt just as confused and worried the day someone said, "These CO_2s are too high. They have to be brought down." What would happen if they didn't come down?

Another time, a resident walked by David, looked at him, shook her head, and walked away. I don't know what that meant, but it worried me for days.

In the beginning, my husband and I were afraid to ask these questions that bothered us. Then one day a nurse gave us some advice. She said that if we weren't ready to ask questions, it was because we weren't ready to hear the answers. It wasn't until then that we realized just how many questions we had been afraid to ask. We had concentrated so long on the condition of David's lungs; I guess we convinced ourselves that if his lungs improved, everything else would be fine. When we realized that this might not be the case, we knew we'd soon have to start asking questions. My first chance came a little while later when a nurse who was massaging David told me that the stiffness in his arms and legs was a sign of hypertonia. When I went home, I looked up the term and found the sentence that read, "This can be an early sign of cerebral palsy." I read and reread that sentence over and over again. Then I had to decide if I was ready to hear the answer if I asked the doctor the question. When the developmental pediatrician came into the nursery later that week, I decided to ask him if David was at risk for developing this disability. Although he couldn't completely rule out that possibility, he believed that with a little physical therapy David would be all right. This wasn't the guarantee I had hoped for, but at least I knew the facts and I was starting to learn that no one can fully predict what will happen in a preemie's future.

Setbacks, whether labeled "big" or "small" by the doctors, were always major to us. No matter what kind of complication developed, we always wondered if this would be the illness that would take our child's life. The setback that was the hardest for us to deal with was when David was put back on the respirator after he had been off it for a month. David had developed something, I'm not even sure now what it was, but he had a bad reaction to the drug that was used to treat the problem, and once again he needed help to keep up a steady breathing pattern. After having come from the respirator, to CPAP, to the oxygen hood, to a cannula, it was so hard to see him back where he was on the first day. It was like starting all over again. Although the neonatologist told us that David's problem wasn't life-threatening, we were still disappointed and worried about what could happen next. I kept thinking, "How much more can this little person endure? How much longer can he fight back?"

Over the course of the next few weeks, David actually improved. He graduated (again) to the oxygen hood and then to the cannula. After that, slowly he began to show more obvious signs of improvement. The IV lines were removed; he was fed by NG tube and bottle; he was introduced to cereal and prune juice, and he began to gain weight. His eyes were examined, and as far as the ophthalmologist could tell at that point, they were fine. Very slowly David was becoming our son, rather than their patient.

Now we were taking on more and more responsibility for David's care. We were able to change his diaper, and tube- and nipple-feed him. We learned how to take his temperature, bathe him, give him his chest physiotherapy, and suction mucus from his nose and mouth. We were taught how to use a stethoscope, how to administer CPR, and how to count David's respirations. We learned these things a little at a time through the patient guidance of the nurses, doctors, and respiratory therapists. Whenever it seemed like we were comfortable with one skill, they'd ask us if we'd like to do something more. In this way, David's care was slowly transferred from their hands to ours.

Quite unexpectedly, the next setback was mine. It happened after I spent my first full day parenting David. From eleven o'clock in the morning until four o'clock in the afternoon I did everything for him. I took his temperature, changed his diapers, administered his chest physiotherapy, gave him a bath, fed him, rocked him, cuddled him, and loved him. That night was the first time in two months that I was just too tired to go back for the evening shift. The next morning the reason for my tiredness showed in small red spots on my back and chest. I had the chicken pox! I couldn't believe it; I had taught grammar school for nine years without catching them, and now with my son in an incubator to isolate him from germs, and right after my first day of prolonged direct exposure to him, I come down with a contagious disease. I was more sick with worry than with the virus. If David caught it, he could develop pneumonia. And what about all the other babies in the nursery? I had endangered their health as well. The next week passed slowly as I waited to see what would happen. Miraculously, none of the babies caught the chicken pox from me.

For three months the ICN was our home, and all the people in it became our adopted family. In the beginning we felt that the nurses, doctors, and therapists existed only for us; we hardly noticed that there were other babies and parents in the nursery. I guess it was a self-centered reaction, but we didn't want to know about anybody else's problems. We were only concerned with David. But as time went on, especially since we were both there every day, we began to become aware of the other families. Small conversations would start up and these eventually led to friendships and a central core of support. While critical health care procedures and important decisions were being handled all around us, we would look to each other for encouragement and even an occasional laugh. The ICN parents would lightheartedly ask each other if the baby had passed what we called the "water test." This measured his ability to hold down a feeding of water. If the baby did that successfully, he advanced to formula; if not, he went back on the IV. We also joked about the babies' hairstyles. Many of them came into the nursery with full heads of hair, but when the ICN "barber" finished placing the scalp IVs, some would sport the "Mr. T" look, others took on a "Telly Savalas" shine, and there were quite a few boys and girls vying for the "Cyndi Lauper" look-alike award. These ICN parents, the health care professionals, and our own immediate family understood what we were going through. When we prayed for our David, we also said a prayer of thanks for all the people who helped pull us through that very difficult time.

Three months and two days, and one hundred thousand dollars later, David (now weighing 7 pounds 12 ounces) was ready to be discharged. George and I were overjoyed at the thought of bringing David home, but we were also a little anxious. This uncertainty was eased a great deal, however, after we both stayed one night with David three days before his release from the hospital. The three of us were given our own room. David was completely under our care, and although the ICN was only forty feet away, this trial run gave us a feeling of independence and confidence.

Before bringing David home, we made preparations for his medical care. Because he had developed BPD (bronchopulmonary dysplasia) he still needed supplemental oxygen. We rented an oxygen concentrator. (This machine takes in room air and converts it to pure oxygen. A small bubble humidifier is attached to the concentrator to moisturize the oxygenated air.) Because our home is a colonial with bedrooms upstairs, the concentrator was strategically placed downstairs in our living room. A hole about ½ inch in diameter was drilled through the ceiling in our living room and into our bedroom where David's crib was located. One end of a 25-foot-long plastic tube about ¼ inch in diameter was attached to the concentrator's humidifier, and the other end was threaded through the hole in the ceiling to David's crib. Another hose was run from the concentrator to David's downstairs crib. Having a separate hose for each level of the house made taking care of David a little easier since he needed supplemental oxygen around the clock for the first eight months at home, and then during the night until he was two years old.

We also rented a pediatric hand resuscitator (in case David stopped breathing), a chest percussor for David's chest physiotherapy, and a portable oxygen unit to use whenever we left the house. (We took David out during his first year and a half only for medical checkups. Because he had BPD he could not go out into crowds for fear of catching a cold, which in his case could lead to pneumonia.)

Then we prepared for possible emergency situations. Because the concentrator ran on electricity, the electric company that services our area was notified. Although we were equipped with a portable unit, it provided oxygen for only about twelve hours when it was full. Therefore, it there was a power outage in our town, the electric company would know that we needed electricity restored immediately. We also notified our town police and ambulance squad of our situation in case we needed their assistance. We posted the phone numbers of the intensive care nursery, the doctors, and the ambulance squad by our phone. And although we had learned CPR at the hospital, we took the CPR course given by the local Red Cross, too. We thought we were ready for David's homecoming, but looking back now, we realize we had no idea how much time David's care would require.

At each feeding David could hold down only 50 cc of formula mixed with two teaspoons of cereal. Therefore, he had to be fed about every three to four hours around the clock. Chest physiotherapy had to be administered three to four times throughout the day to keep his lungs clear. These rhythmic "tappings" on his back had to be scheduled at least one hour before or after feedings to prevent regurgitation. David's physical therapy exercises (which totaled from one half to one full hour each day) were given in ten- to fifteen-minute sessions. In addition, the concentrator hose and humidifier had to be cleaned daily. (David was put on the portable unit while this was done.) The concentrator hose would accumulate moisture, which could go into the baby's nose, or even worse, his lungs. To prevent bacterial growth, the humidifier had to be washed with vinegar and water. We made new cannulas every few days or so, depending on how dirty they became. David's medication schedule required very careful planning. He was given Lasix at 9 A.M. to keep his lungs clear, vitamins at noon, phenobarbital to prevent seizures at 6 A.M. and P.M., and nystatin for thrush at 9 A.M. and P.M. Add to all this the routine care of a baby and normal household duties, and our days were quite full.

For the first eight months we went to the neonatologist for checkups. At first we went weekly, then biweekly, then monthly, until David was put under the pediatrician's care. During this time he also needed to see a physical therapist. The muscles in his arms and legs were still stiff, and his shoulders and arms had a tendency to move back away from his chest rather than to fall forward. This therapy began on a weekly basis, and then was given biweekly until he was discharged by the therapist when he was thirteen months old. He was also routinely checked by a developmental pediatrician and a developmental psychologist.

When I look back now, I marvel that George and I were able to get through those first few years. I guess because David was our first child, his exceptional care needs seemed normal to us. And because he was our only child, we had the time to devote ourselves entirely to him. During the first year I spent *all* my time at home caring for David. The only time I was away from him was while his grandparents babysat and I went grocery shopping on Friday mornings and to church on Sundays. Although I led a secluded life at that time, I really didn't mind; I think I even enjoyed it. There was always so much to do to care for David, and I felt so much happiness after a good checkup and when he showed improvement at the physical therapy sessions—that was all I needed to keep going. I also think that when it comes to your own child, there's no such thing as, "I can't do it." You do what you have to do.

Today, David is four years old, weighs thirty pounds, and is forty inches tall. His health is good and he attends nursery school with his friends two days a week. Now, he is just like every other child his age—so much so that sometimes we forget how difficult things were at the start. Preparing this story has been therapeutic for George and me because we shared feelings and thoughts that we had never before discussed. At the time of David's birth and hospitalization it was sometimes hard to share our pain, but looking back as we write this, we've come to realize that there were three common factors that helped both of us keep going: We both loved our son; We trusted David's doctors; and we had our religious faith.

Prayers became an important part of our time in the ICN. We believed in the power of God and in His mercy, and we both prayed every day for David's recovery. We now realize that even our initial prayers for the delivery of a healthy baby have been answered—maybe a little later than we would have liked—because we do have a very healthy little boy at last.

Chapter Six

. . . .

Moderately Premature Babies*

35 to 37 Weeks Gestational Age

Babies who are born at 35 to 37 weeks gestational age (3 to 5 weeks early) are called moderately premature.* Most often these babies weigh between 1701 and 3402 grams about (3 pounds 12 ounces to 7 pounds 8 ounces), and are, on average, 17 to 18 inches long. The survival rate for these babies is 98 to 100 percent.†

*All terms and medical procedures mentioned in this chapter have been explained in detail in other parts of the book, or are defined in the Glossary. Use the cross-references or the Index to find the pages that give more detailed information.

†This statistic excludes those babies born with the kinds of birth defects that are not directly related to prematurity. Defects such as chromosomal abnormalities, or severe heart or brain defects also affect the survival rates of full-term infants.

PHYSICAL APPEARANCE

Although the moderately premature baby is only 3 to 5 weeks from term, in physical appearance he is obviously still immature. Since a fetus will gain approximately a half pound during each of the last 5 weeks in utero, the baby born even a bit too soon comes into the world lacking a large percentage of his relative full-term weight. He is also often at a disadvantage in his ability to self-regulate his body systems. For these reasons, even the moderately premature child requires immediate attention, evaluation, and guarded monitoring at birth.

Next to the younger preemie, however, this baby who has had the advantage of extra weeks in the nurturing environment of his mother's uterus, certainly appears more "full grown." He has more body fat than the very or very-very premature baby, and so he appears sturdier and stronger. Also, his skin is thicker and it has lost the translucent appearance common in younger preemies. He has less body and facial hair (called lanugo), and he has better muscle tone that now enables him to tuck in his arms and legs in the normal fetal position. The moderately premature baby has enough cartilage in his ears so that if an ear is folded down, it will spring back into shape, and he has thicker, and more fully shaped fingernails. The eyelids are fully matured, and the eyelashes are fully grown. A baby boy's testes have descended into the scrotum, and a baby girl's outer vaginal tissues are beginning to cover the clitoris fully.

BODY TEMPERATURE CONTROL

Even though the moderately premature baby has more body fat than younger preemies, he still may not be able to regulate his own body temperature. If he needs artificial warmth, either he will be placed in an incubator, or he will wear a cap and be wrapped in extra blankets. A few babies, who are sufficiently plump, can be cared for in open bassinets.

RESPIRATORY CARE

Eighty to ninety percent of moderately premature babies have fully matured lungs. Some of these babies instantaneously breathe on their own and require no respiratory aid. Others may need minimal respiratory assistance and are given extra oxygen and humidity through the tube of an oxygen hood. Only a small number of these preemies need the more intensive therapy supplied through CPAP or a respirator.

Initial respiratory distress may be caused by scheduled and/or elective cesarean deliveries. This sometimes happens because these C-section babies do not have the benefit of the uterine contractions that push on their thorax and rid them of the excess fluid that collects in the chest cavity. The resultant respiratory problems usually improve after twelve to twenty-four hours on IV fluids and respiratory support systems.

It is unusual for mildly premature infants to experience apnea and/or bradycardia episodes after 34 weeks gestational age. At this time the lungs are usually mature enough to give the baby control of his respiratory patterns. However, a preemie's respiratory and heart rates (which are generally just a bit faster than those of the full-term baby) are routinely monitored for the first few days after birth with the electrodes and wires described in Chapter Two. Therefore, if the baby should experience a breathing pause or an increased or decreased heartbeat, the doctors and nurses will be immediately alerted to the problem.

FEEDING METHODS

It is unlikely that a mother will be able to breast-feed her moderately premature baby in the delivery room immediately after birth. When a baby is born prematurely, he is immediately taken to a radiant warmer to ensure adequate warmth, and his vital signs are promptly stabilized and monitored. Once the doctors have finished this exam and evaluation, they will be able to assess the baby's ability to suck, swallow, and breathe in a coordinated manner. They can then decide on the best approach to feeding.

Some moderately premature babies are not yet ready for bottle- or breast-feeding. (This is especially true of preemies experiencing respiratory difficulties. Oral feedings are introduced only after the respiratory system is stable.) These babies will be fed formula or breast milk through an NG tube or with a special bottle nipple that doesn't require such strenuous sucking. (A small number of these preemies may have digestive difficulties and will therefore be fed parenteral solution initially through an IV. The majority of moderately premature babies, however, are able to suck well enough to be bottle- or breast-fed.) If the baby's sucking is not vigorous enough to guarantee necessary fluid and nutrient intake, these feedings will be supplemented with NG tube feedings of breast milk or formula. (If your breast-feedings are supplemented or delayed, be sure to pump your breast milk every day to stimulate the let-down reflex and to ensure an ample supply when your baby is ready.)

BEHAVIOR

Babies who are born 3 to 5 weeks prematurely have a better-developed central nervous system than younger premature babies. This enables them to sleep peacefully for longer periods of time because they are less irritable and hyperreactive to stimulation. These babies are also more easily soothed by the feel of your touch and the sound of your voice.

The moderately premature baby is gaining in muscle strength. His arm and leg movements are now smoother and more purposeful, and the baby may move them in back-and-forth alternating patterns. Many moderately premature babies may also be able to bring their hands to their mouths, and can make an effort to hold their heads up when pulled to a sitting position. When supported in a sitting position, many can lift their heads off the chest and remain upright for several seconds. At 37 weeks the hand-grasp reflex and upper arm muscles are strong enough to allow these babies to hold tight while they are pulled up to a sitting position.

These older preemies can see almost as well as full-term babies. They will turn their eyes to a soft light. They will begin to exhibit a distinct preference for patterns (particularly those with a greater number of large details). They may also prefer curved lines over straight lines in pictures.

TRANSFER INFORMATION

Most babies born at this stage of prematurity do not need intensive care. Often a pediatrician can competently care for these babies, and the facilities at the Level I and II hospitals are fully equipped to give them appropriate attention. Therefore, a moderately premature baby will not be transferred to a higher-level care facililty unless (as is the case with any newborn) he has health complications, such as breathing or feeding difficulties, that require exceptional medical intervention. However, moderately premature babies do need extra attention and time to grow, so their stay in the hospital will often be one to two weeks longer than that of a full-term baby.

PARENTING TIPS

Like all newborns, your moderately premature baby needs lots of sleep to grow in size and strength. But unlike younger premature infants, he will probably have extended awake periods each day. Some babies may have predictable periods during which they can stay awake for as long as thirty minutes. (Ask the nurses if they've noticed a wake/sleep pattern. They sometimes keep a record of sleep cycles.) If you can guess when your baby will be awake, try to arrange your visits around that schedule. It's not a good idea to wake a sleeping preemie just to say hello. But if he's already awake, this is a good opportunity to get acquainted.

If the doctor says your baby is ready for bottle- or breast-feedings, this is usually a good time to help him practice. Because oral feedings will tire even a moderately premature baby, it is usually best not to overstimulate him by also talking, smiling, singing, or trying to make eye contact while he's feeding. Sit back, relax, and follow the tips on oral feeding given in Chapter Eight.

If your baby is able to come out of the incubator, use some of his awake time for holding and rocking him. As you sit back in the chair and hold your baby close to your chest, you may see him trying to lift his head to look at you. If you hold him up over your shoulder, he may also lift his head and turn his face to see yours. This is a good indication that he is ready for some visual stimulation. Although he does not have complete or clear vision, his ability to focus on and follow your face or a brightly colored object is rapidly developing. As long as he's not trying to feed, hold your baby in a face-to-face position (about eight to twelve inches away from you) and talk or sing to him and smile. Once you see him focusing on you, move your face slowly from side to side, then up and down. He will gradually learn to follow you. If you lose your baby's attention, just start again. You can also practice this exercise with a brightly colored object or toy. For the times you can't be with your baby, or if he can't yet come out of the incubator, you can provide him with visual stimulation by placing one or two brightly colored toys next to him. See Chapter Eight for incubator-decorating ideas.

As you spend awake time with your baby, watch for signs of discomfort or tiredness. Moderately premature babies are able to express displeasure by crying, but many may still show signs of fatigue or overstimulation by changes in their behavior. Some may say it's time-to-stop through changes in their color or rate of respiration, others by yawning, sneezing, or hiccupping, or you may notice your baby start to fuss and squirm. As much as you might want to continue holding or playing with your baby, when he signals that he's had enough, give him a kiss and put him back in his bed until he's rested and ready to try again.

Alycia's and Virginia's Story

by Lisa Crilly

I had a good pregnancy with no complications at all. I knew from a sonogram that I was going to have twins, and I knew from my experience as a physical therapist working with children in hospitals that there was a good chance the babies could be born early. I always thought if that happened, I'd have no trouble dealing with it because I had been trained to understand the developmental process involved in working with premature babies. But as soon as my babies were born, all my professional training took a backseat to my emotions. Now I wasn't the therapist; I was the mom, and all I had to work with were my emotions and my gut feelings.

My girls were born on January 4, 1988, at 35 weeks gestational age. I had a relatively easy three-hour labor and then a natural, vaginal delivery. Alycia was born first and she weighed 4 pounds 5 ounces. Then eleven minutes later, Virginia arrived weighing 4 pounds 11 ounces. My first question was, "Are they healthy?" Although I didn't get to see for myself right away, the neonatologist was very optimistic. He said the babies were healthy, but they were small and had a few minor problems, so they would be kept in the special nursery. The first time I saw them in this special nursery, it was hard for me to feel as optimistic as everyone else there who kept telling me they were doing very well.

Both girls were in incubators because they didn't have enough body fat of their own. Each one had a black wire attached to a foot (it was held in place with wrapped gauze) that monitored the body oxygen. Because they were having trouble digesting food and they weren't strong enough yet to suck on a bottle nipple, each one was being fed through an IV tube inserted into a vein in an arm. Gina had

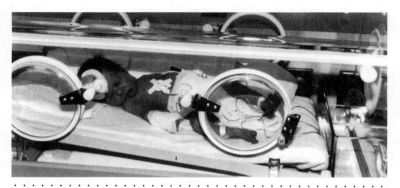

Alycia at two days

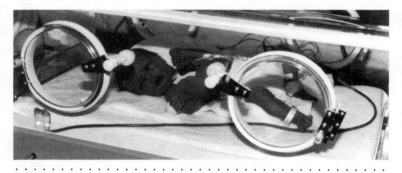

Virginia at two days

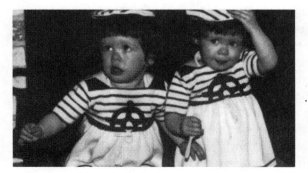

*Alycia and
Virginia,
seventeen
months*

an NG tube placed through her nose to suction excess mucus from her stomach. They both had jaundice so they were wearing goggles and had bililights over them. And they also were attached to the wires that monitored the heart and breathing rates. So there lay my "healthy" babies looking to me like they'd never live through the day. No matter how many times I told myself, "Your babies are fine; they're going to be okay," I would look at these sweet little children, all entangled in medical equipment, and just cry.

I didn't think it could be possible, but the next day Gina looked even worse. Apparently, she didn't like all those tubes and wires so she kept trying to pull them out. The nurses put her arms in wrist restraints, but she always managed to get out of them. (We gave her the nickname "Houdini.") Because she kept pulling out the IV, the little veins in her wrists and arms collapsed, so they had to put the IV into a vein in her scalp. Now, not only did she have the heart and breathing monitors, the NG tube, and the wrist restraints, but her head was almost completely shaved and she had an IV line going into her head that was held in place with strips of tape.

It was so hard for me to stand by the incubators every day, look at my babies like this, and not be able to comfort or hold them. All I could do for the first four days was put my hand through the porthole and pet them. My maternal drive was so strong at that time, but I couldn't use it. I couldn't cradle my babies in my arms; I couldn't feed them or nurture them. Now I'm embarrassed to admit it, but at the time I felt both anger and jealousy when I saw the other mothers whose babies were in the regular nursery. All through the day and night, I'd hear the little cribs being wheeled around to their mothers' beds so they could be held and fed. Sometimes at feeding times, I'd put on my robe and go into the special nursery just to sit next to my babies. This was the time I was supposed to be with them. Then I'd go back to my room and feel the most awful guilt I've ever known. I'd picture in my mind all those tubes and wires, and I'd think how confused and afraid my babies must be. I thought I should be the one suffering because it was my fault that they were born prematurely. The week before their birth, I was taking down the Christmas tree and my husband Jack said to me, "You shouldn't be reaching and bending like that. You should take it easy." I just brushed him off and said, "Oh, stop it. I'm fine." Lying in that hospital bed without my babies in my arms, I was so angry at myself. Over and over I'd say, "You should have been more careful. You should have thought more about your responsibility to the babies. It's your fault you went into premature labor." Today I know that what happened was the way it was meant to be and no one is to blame. But at the time, I was convinced that I had personally caused every problem and discomfort my children had to bear.

Feeding time became the focus of my days because I knew the twins couldn't go home until they gained weight. The nurses would weigh the girls every day, and every day I'd run in and ask, "How much did they gain?" In the beginning, it was never good news. Alycia went down from 4 pounds 5 ounces to 4 pounds 4 ounces, to 3 ounces, to 2, to 1 and then to a flat 4 pounds. Gina was doing the same. I kept thinking, "When are they going to grow?" The growing process was so slow. I remember one day, I came into the nursery, and a nurse told me that Gina had taken all her formula. For the first time since their birth, I felt elated. Then I looked into her incubator and saw that she had spit up the whole feeding. At that point I think I honestly believed they were never going to get bigger.

The girls fed every three hours. When the nurses began feeding them formula from a bottle, I was still in the hospital and I watched them very carefully so I could begin feeding them myself. We tried to juggle their feeding times so that Jack and I could hold them and try to feed them a few times each day. We tried so hard, but it was very discouraging in the beginning because their sucking reflexes were still so weak. After almost an hour of trying to feed them, we'd see that they had taken only about half the amount they were supposed to, but we'd patiently keep trying. One day a nurse told us (as nicely as she could), that although we were doing a good job, when the babies take that long to feed, they burn more calories trying to suck than they take in as formula. Jack and I looked at each other with the same thought: "These babies will never get out of this hospital."

The first one to go home was me. I still get a lump in my throat and my eyes fill up with tears when I think about walking out of that hospital without my babies. I said goodbye to them; then I called Jack and told him to come and get me right away. Even though I didn't want to go home, I knew the longer I stayed, the more difficult it would be to leave. There was a snowstorm that day, so it took a long time for Jack to get to the hospital. When I was waiting, I kept saying to myself, "He's got to come now because I don't want to go back and say good-bye again." Finally, he came. We went right past the nursery, out to the parking lot, and then I cried for the entire thirty-minute ride home. I had gone into that hospital with two babies cradled safely inside of me, and now I was going home with none. We weren't home even five minutes when I told Jack I wanted to go back to the hospital. He must have felt the same way because he didn't even give me one of those "Are you crazy?" looks. We went right out to the car and headed back through the snowstorm to begin our days of outpatient visiting.

I was worried about how well I could bond with the girls; there seemed to be so many obstacles in our way. At first I thought it would be impossible because I couldn't even hold them in my arms. Then when I did, it was awkward and uncomfortable because of all the wires and tubes.

Also, because there were two of them, I had to share my time back and forth between incubators. Now I was going to be living twenty-five miles away from them. I guess that's why it was so important to me to spend as much time with them as I could. Jack had to work, but he'd drop me off at the hospital about six-thirty each morning so I could be there for the first feeding, and I'd stay until Jack came back at seven each night. Then the two of us would feed them and go home.

I don't think the babies' health improved just because I was there every day, but sometimes I felt like my presence could safeguard them against complications, and the more I could look at them and hold them, the better we would bond. I'm not surely exactly how or when it happened, but despite the problems of trying to be good parents in a crowded room where everybody else knew more about our babies than we did, I know that no other parents have ever bonded more closely or felt more love for a baby than Jack and I feel for our Alycia and Gina. That's why we wanted them to come home with us. We worried so often that they would never get bigger and stronger. But they did.

We agonized through two weeks of up-and-down reports from doctors and nurses: "Her bilirubin count is okay, we can take away the bililights; oops, it went up again, so we're bringing back the lamps." "The IV can come out today; oops, we had to put one back in." "She gained half an ounce today; oops, she's lost another ounce." After screaming in my heart a hundred times, "Will this ever end?!" they finally started to grow. When their weight began to go up steadily, first the IVs came out for good. Then, one-by-one, the breathing and heart monitors disappeared, the NG tube was gone, the eye goggles were put away, and the bililight was removed. One morning, I went into the nursery and saw my babies lying in their incubators without any medical things around them. All I saw were two little girls—two normal children who looked beautiful. They still showed some battle scars (Gina's head was still shaved, and she had red tape marks all over her face from where the NG tube was held in place, and also on her forehead from the IV), but the nurses said the marks wouldn't last long. And they were right; when I came back for the very next feeding they already looked much better.

One day shortly after that, the neonatologist said, "Let's try them in a crib." They were still in the special nursery, but they were on their own. Now I had no doubt that they really would be coming home soon. As I was sitting in the corner by their new cribs, Jack came in on his lunch hour for a quick visit. He went over to the incubator where Gina had been. I guess preemies tend to look somewhat alike, and so he stood there staring at this baby thinking she was Gina. This little baby must have just had chest surgery because she had a scar running down the length of her body. Jack turned white as a sheet. I walked over and tried to pull him away to tell him that Gina had been moved, but he wouldn't look at me. His eyes were full of tears, and all he kept saying was, "Why didn't you tell me this happened? You didn't even call me." This experience made us realize how lucky we really were, and it also made us feel a great deal of empathy for all the other babies in the nursery and all their parents. Each one had his own special problems; each one, like us, was emotionally braced for the setback that could happen at any moment.

The babies continued to do fine after they came out of the incubator. They were holding a good body temperature, and their weight was still slowly but gradually increasing. Two days later the neonatologist asked me if I would like to take Alycia home the next day. At first I was thrilled; I couldn't believe I could really have my baby at home. But then I realized he had mentioned only one of them. The doctor must have seen my face fall and the tears start to come when I asked him, "What about Gina?" So he smiled and said, "What if I let both of them go home in two days?" I'd waited so long to hear those words; now they sounded too good to be true.

I went down to the lobby and got about a hundred dimes and called everyone I knew to tell them my babies were coming home. No one had seen my babies (except my parents, who were allowed grandparent visits). My other relatives, friends, and neighbors only saw pictures. It had made me sad to say, "I have two beautiful baby girls, but you can't see them yet." One of the happiest things you can do in life is to bring home a newborn and say, "Look, this is my baby." Now it was finally our turn to do that. All the time of worrying and wondering "Will they ever get bigger? Will they ever be able to come home?" was over. Two weeks after their birth, weighing 4 pounds 2 ounces, and 4 pounds 6 ounces, they were coming home.

When we got home I found out that the two weeks of hospital parenting really had been a blessing in disguise. I had had a chance to learn so much from the neonatologist and the nurses. I watched every move they made, and they patiently explained everything they did. I felt like I had had private training in how to care for premature children. By the time we got home, Jack and I weren't at all afraid to handle or care for our babies. I felt like every question I could possibly have had already been answered. (It was my mother and sister who needed a lot of coaching before they could comfortably handle the babies!)

After I was home for a while, I realized how exceptionally wonderful everyone in the hospital had been to all of us. I could call in the middle of the night and never have to worry that I was bothering them. I never felt like I was in their way when I sat by the incubators, and they never made me fell incompetent when I asked what probably were silly questions. I doubt these people will ever really know how much their skill, knowledge, and compassion mean to the parents of the preemies they care for. Without a second thought, I trusted them with a part of me. There is no way to say "Thanks" for that. I just hope somehow they know how grateful we are.

The follow-up examinations have all gone very well. We went for our first pediatric checkup one week after the babies came home. At three weeks of age, Alycia weighed almost 5 pounds and Gina weighed just a bit more. I came home and again ran to the telephone. I called my husband, my parents, my friends, and even the neonatologist and the nurses at the hospital. I was so excited that the babies had grown so big and that everything was really going to be fine.

The girls continued to do well at their regular checkups, and they went back to the neonatologist when they were four months and twelve months old for general neurological and developmental evaluations. I had been videotapping their progress once a month for my own sake, and for my professional interest, and I was watching closely for any abnormal growth patterns. Even though I knew all about developmental progress from my work as a therapist, I still had to keep reminding myself to consider the corrected age not the birth age. Sometimes they were right on schedule, other times they were slower to catch up and I'd start to worry. Of course, in the long run, it didn't really matter if they rolled over or sat up on the exact day I thought they should, as long as they were generally on target and growing stronger each day.

Alycia and Gina both have grown into beautiful, healthy, normal children. When I look back over their first year, I know it was, all at the same time, the scariest, saddest, happiest, and most exciting time of my life.

Chapter Seven

. . . .

Facing Your Feelings

There is a lot to learn about your premature baby. He lives in a world filled with unfamiliar statistical data, complex equipment, unending testing procedures, and confusing medical complications that are all supervised by a battalion of caretakers who talk in an abbreviated language resembling alphabet soup. It's no wonder that with so much to learn, so much to worry about, and with such an intense focus on *the baby,* your own feelings, as well as your relationship with your spouse and your other children, may be ignored.

Try not to slight your own needs and feelings. Even while your baby is in the hospital, you deserve attention, and you need time for yourself and your family. Taking care of yourself and learning how to accept what you're feeling isn't a selfish act; it's an absolutely necessary step you have to take before you can lovingly care for your baby.

Each parent has his or her own personal way of reacting to the premature birth of a baby. Some cry all the time; some don't cry at all. Some want to be with the baby every second; some can't bring themselves even to look at the child. The only element that is common to all parents in this situation is the fact that whatever they feel about the birth at any given moment is okay. For most parents of preemies, the first year of the baby's life is an emotional roller coaster. There are moments of great joy, happiness, and relief that are sure to plummet to the depths of disappointment, guilt, and depression, and then rise and fall again. Give yourself permission to accept the angry, hateful feelings as well as the pride and hope.

Although the vast majority of preemies go on to live healthy, normal lives, the initial uncertainty of each day's prognosis can certainly cause you to feel many different emotions. No two parents will ever feel exactly the same way or pass through the same stages of acceptance at the same time, but there are a group of feelings that many parents commonly experience after the birth of their baby. These include: shock, panic, denial, anger, and sadness; and deep down, mixed among these is an underlying sense of hope.

Your feelings may run the gamut of all of these, or you may find yourself stuck in one. Each one is discussed in this chapter in the belief that seeing the secrets of your heart written down in black and white, and expressed openly by other parents will help you realize that what you're feeling is normal, and that you're not alone on this emotional roller coaster.

SHOCK

Just as the body may go into shock when it is overwhelmed by a physical trauma, some parents go into emotional shock when they are confronted with a traumatic situation. If you often feel numb and detached and have periods of apathy, incoherence, and unresponsiveness, you may be in a state of shock. You may even experience physical reactions such as pale, moist, clammy skin; general weakness; a rapid, weak pulse; and/or fast, shallow, and irregular breathing that sometimes may be accompanied by nausea and/or loss of appetite.

Two years after the premature birth of her son, Susan still remembers very clearly how she felt when he was transferred to another hospital to be treated for pneumonia. "Brian was two days old when he developed pneumonia. I remember that I had just started to accept the fact that he was born so early, and I was just starting to recover from the difficult delivery when the pediatrician came into my hospital room with a somber look on his face. When he first told me that Brian had pneumonia, it didn't sound like anything to look so concerned about—lots of people get pneumonia. But when he told me that Brian was being transferred to an intensive care nursery because in preemies this infection could cause other serious complications and could be fatal, I went into shock. I just sat there staring at my hands. The doctor kept talking and he kept asking me if I understood, but I couldn't talk back. It was like my mind just froze. I couldn't go back and think about what he had just said, and I couldn't go forward to think about the arrangements that were being made to move my baby. It was like I was trapped in this awful place where I couldn't cry, or move, or talk. Although people were on the outside trying to make me respond, I just couldn't let them in to help me. I spent the next three or four days like that. As soon as I was discharged from the hospital, I went to Brian's new nursery and I sat by his incubator all day every day without seeing or hearing anyone else in the room. I felt like my mind, my emotions, my whole being was still locked back in that moment when the pediatrician told me Brian could die.

"Finally one night when I came home from the hospital and again went straight to bed without even saying good-

night, my husband gave up trying to be patient and understanding with me. He started yelling at me; I could hear the
pain in his voice but I still couldn't respond. He begged me
to help him understand how I was feeling. He said he
could't stand being shut out anymore and he wanted to
face this together. I just stared at him. Suddenly he grabbed
me by the shoulders, pulled me up off the bed, and threw
his arms around me and cried—then I started to cry. We
both stood there sobbing in each other's arms. I don't really know how or why, but as he wiped my tears away, I
felt much better and I was ready to move on and deal with
my baby's medical problems."

PANIC

The first rule in an emergency is "Don't panic." This is
because in a state of panic, it's impossible to act in an organized, rational, or efficient manner. When you first hear
that your baby's health may be in danger, you may panic
and lose control of the situation. In this state you may become overwhelmed and react with feelings of anxiety,
helplessness, or hysteria.

Joe's preemie is still in the hospital and is still struggling
to overcome some serious setbacks, but already he can look
back and recognize a time of pure panic. "I always thought
that panic was a momentary reaction to something catastrophic, but now I know that's not necessarily how it
works. Right after Ashley's birth, I spent at least two full
weeks in the state of panic. I felt like a caged wild animal
crashing back and forth against the bars because I couldn't
do anything constructive about the situation. I found it very
difficult to do even the most routine things. I couldn't decide what to wear, or what to eat, or when to visit the
nursery, or what to ask the doctors, or what to say to my
wife. Everything seemed too overwhelming to deal with.

"I'm surprised I didn't lose my job during that time. I became so disorganized that the top of my desk looked like the aftermath of a tornado. I couldn't find a thing; I couldn't remember what I was looking for; and I couldn't sit still long enough to do the work even if I found it. I also became very forgetful. I'd miss important appointments, forget my briefcase at home, and ignore deadlines. Then, when I'd made a big enough mess of things, I'd snap at anyone who'd even look at me funny.

"I don't know what brought me out of it (I can't even say for sure that I'm in complete control now), but I think that once the mind has a chance to absorb all the medical stuff that goes with a premature birth, then that awful, helpless feeling gradually subsides. I know in my case, when I finally understood what all the tubes and wires and medical procedures were all about, I was finally able to put my own life back in order."

DENIAL

Denial is a very common emotional state in adults with a terminal disease. They may insist, "That doctor doesn't know what he's talking about. I feel just fine." These people may refuse to talk about their illness; they may ignore the doctor's instructions, and they may refuse to make final personal and financial decisions. Just as it is difficult to accept our own mortality, it may be difficult for you to accept the birth of a baby who is less than plump, happy, and healthy. It's hard to say how long you might go on denying the state of your baby's health, but almost always the reality of the situation will sink in when you are emotionally ready to handle it.

Both Jane and Randy experienced emotional denial after the premature birth of their child, yet they expressed it in very different ways. "In the beginning," says Jane, "I wouldn't let myself consider the possibility that Jennifer wasn't just fine. If she had a few problems, I knew that somebody somewhere could fix them. If Jennifer's doctors said anything I didn't want to hear, I immediately set out to find a specialist who could give me a second opinion that sounded more positive. If no one would tell me what I wanted to hear, I'd go to sleep; I guess this was a way for me to escape from a situation I didn't want to face. Sometimes when I'd first wake up, there'd be a split second when I'd forget that Jennifer had been born. For that fraction of a moment I'd feel calm; then I'd remember, and that chill inside of me would come back.

"For all the sleeping I did, I never really felt rested and I began to look and feel run-down. I found denial to be very exhausting. I think it was fatigue that finally made me break down and agree to listen to the facts as they really were. At this point I was ready to talk about Jennifer's health, and that's when I noticed that Randy had found his own way to avoid facing the truth.

"Randy had become so busy at work that he didn't have time to think about Jennifer. All of a sudden he had to work very late every night so, of course, he didn't have time to visit the nursery. He also didn't have the time to talk to me about our child, and he certainly didn't have time to listen to the doctors explain what they were doing to save Jennifer's life. At the time, I really think he believed that the work just piled up at this inopportune time, and it had nothing to do with his feelings for his daughter. His sudden "too busy" mentality wasn't a devious plan to ignore what was going on; I think it was a subconscious thing he did to protect himself from facing the pain he felt about having a sick child. Unfortunately, his protective shield came between the two of us.

"For months after Jennifer's birth we never went anywhere socially; we very rarely even talked to each other. I don't understand how this happened because before this we were very close and loving. Maybe we were afraid that opening up to each other would bring out the truth and bring in the pain we were both trying to avoid. Anyway, we still haven't been able to get our relationship back to where it was before the baby. I wish we were able to find some way to pull together and help each other during this time, but we can't. Maybe now that Jennifer is ready to come home, Randy and I will be able to work on our feelings for each other. I hope so.''

ANGER

Before the birth of your preemie, what kinds of things made you really angry—the kind of spitting-mad angry that caused you to kick walls and throw things? Most people feel this way when something happens that's absolutely not fair, but that they can't do anything about. That's how you may feel about the early birth of your baby, and it's possible you'll feel this way for a very long time. You may logically know that your baby's early birth is no one's fault, but in your gut you may hate everyone around you, lash out at the doctors and nurses, and say cruel things to anyone who tries to comfort you. Some parents even feel anger toward the baby who turned their lives upside down.

Today Dan realizes that he was actually just angry at the whole situation, but he took it out on the people he loved the most. "My poor family went through hell with me. When little Danny was born 12 weeks early I found myself yelling at everybody who came near me. My parents would say something comforting like "We're sure the baby will be okay," and I'd snap back with something gruff like "How would you know? you don't even know what's wrong with him." If my wife was a little uncertain about what the doctor told her, I'd go into a rage and call her stupid or ignorant or uncaring, or whatever else came out of my mouth in anger. Fortunately for me, my parents and my wife were smart enough to understand my reactions, but I still feel terrible about the way I treated our three-year-old daughter.

"The nine weeks that Danny was in the hospital must have been the hardest on her. I'm sure Kate didn't understand why the new baby couldn't come home, or why her mom and dad didn't have time anymore to play with her. She was shuffled around from babysitter to babysitter, and when she was at home with us, she had to watch her mom crying all the time and listen to me yell at her for every little thing. Sometimes my raised voice would scare her, and she'd run away from me, climb up on her mom's lap, and cry like I'd slapped her across the face. I hated myself for not being more patient with her, but I just felt so angry all the time, I couldn't turn it off even for her. I'm still amazed at how forgiving she was. Every morning she'd act as if nothing had changed; she'd start the day with a smile and give me a big hug. It's going to take some time for me to give back to Kate all the attention and love she missed during that time when Danny was sick, but I'm going to try.

"I'd like right now to say a public 'I'm sorry' to all the people I lashed out at when I hurt too much to let them come close."

SADNESS

No one but a preemie's parent knows the full depth of the sadness that can accompany a premature birth. This sadness can show itself in a wide range of feelings that include guilt, shame, emptiness, and/or depression. Many parents have found that these feelings of sadness are the ones that linger the longest and tend to go and come back again in waves for months, even years, after the baby's birth.

Five years ago, Diane's daughter was born ten weeks early. Even today she cries when she thinks back to those first few months of Kim's life. "In the very beginning, I reacted to Kim's birth with a lot of courage and mental strength. Everyone was surprised that I was holding up so well. Each morning I'd talk with Kim's doctors; I'd ask logical questions; I'd take notes; and then I'd go into the nursery to sit by her incubator and wait for her to grow. Then one afternoon when Kim was about eight days old, I was eating lunch in the park across from the hospital and I saw a mother holding a happy, healthy infant on her lap. It was like reality walked right over and slapped me in the face. I couldn't go back into the hospital; I went straight home, sat in the living room chair, and cried for the rest of the day. I kept thinking, 'Why me? Why my baby?' I started thinking about all the things I did during my pregnancy that might have caused the baby to be born early.

"It took me a long time to get over the guilt and emptiness I felt that day. In fact, some days I didn't even go to see Kim (which made me feel more guilty). It embarrassed me to sit in the nursery crying for no real reason. Compared to some of the other babies, Kim was doing very well, but at that point even good news made me cry. I also thought I looked too awful to go out of the house. I couldn't eat or sleep; I didn't want to fix my hair or put on makeup, and I was too tired to wash or iron clothes. (Now that I think about it, it's probably best that I didn't go out of the house!)

"After the initial plunge into depression, there were some days when I felt better, maybe even optimistic. But then Kim would have a setback, or I'd see a healthy baby somewhere and that awful, empty, sick feeling would start all over again.

"These up-and-down periods must have been hard on my husband. He'd be relieved to see me finally feeling strong and hopeful one day; then the next day, I'd be right back down in the dumps. I know he was worried about Kim, he worried a lot about me, too. When I'd try to choke back tears, he's always say, 'It's okay to cry.' When I was too depressed to go to the hospital, he'd go alone without making me feel ashamed. When I was quiet, he'd just give me a hug. I don't know how I would have made it through those days if Mike weren't so supportive and understanding."

HOPE

Hope is a feeling that for some parents is stronger than all the others. You'll often hear parents of preemies say, "We never gave up hope." Some people call them false hopes; some say it's foolish to be optimistic about prematurity-related complications that are sometimes fatal. But some parents strongly believe their baby will pull through, and they focus on the positive side of the mortality statistics. Hope is what helps them watch the baby go through the ups and downs of prematurity, and keeps them believing that each day is the day their baby will make progress.

For other parents, hope lies deeply hidden beneath all the other emotions and feelings. But almost always, it's there someplace. It's what keeps them coming back to visit their baby even though they're sad, or angry, or in shock. It's the reason why—even as they wonder, "Is all this worth it?" or, "Is it best that this baby lives?"—there is a nagging inner voice that keeps saying "yes."

Considering the wealth of recent technological advances that give premature babies unprecedented hope for a normal, healthy life, you do have good reasons to remain hopeful. However, at the same time, you also have good reasons to feel all the other emotions described in this chapter. Give yourself the freedom to feel whatever comes naturally right now. This will help you move forward until you finally reach the emotional level where you can accept your new life with this child—then you'll be ready to become an involved and caring parent.

There are some things you can do to help yourself reach this stage of acceptance. The list shown offers a few basic ideas.

Suggested Ways to Handle Your Feelings
- Accept your feelings as normal.
- Don't berate yourself for feeling sad or angry.
- Accept other people's reactions as normal for them.
- Allow yourself to delay acceptance of the situation until you're ready.
- Get extra rest and eat nutritious food.
- Let other people help you with daily chores.
- Learn all you can about premature babies.
- Realize that others may not know what to say or how to help you.
- Don't blame yourself or anyone else.
- Expect to feel depressed and tired, and to have good days and not-so-good days.
- When you're ready, talk about your feelings.

All of these things will help quicken your recovery from the shock of having a premature child. Try particularly hard to keep open the lines of communication with your spouse. At first you may worry that talking about your own problems will put more of an emotional burden on your partner. That won't happen. When you talk about your feelings, you'll allow your spouse to open up to and admit his or her own fears and concerns. Both of you are hurting, but you may have different ways of showing it. Talking about it will help you avoid misunderstandings.

Both of you can also find understanding and acceptance from other parents of premature babies. These are the only people who can even begin to know what you're really feeling. Sometimes small talk in the nursery can lead to mutual support and encouragement. You may also find a source of emotional strength in organized parent groups. Ask around to find one in your area. The nurses or the hospital social worker may be able to tell you how to get in touch with one. (Sometimes these groups are sponsored by the hospital.) If you can't find a support group near you (or if you would like to belong to a larger network of parents) call a representative of Parent Care, Inc. (1-703-836-4678). This is a national organization made up of professionals and parents who support the establishment and maintenance of parent support groups in intensive care nurseries. They offer educational brochures, a quarterly newsletter, and a referral service that can put you in touch with a parent support group near you.

In addition, you should be sure to seek the help of family, friends, clergy, and hospital staff members. They are all waiting to give you support when you're ready to accept it.

. . . .

Chapter Eight

Caring for a Preemie

There are many people involved in caring for your premature baby. Chapter Two introduced you to many of these experts and explained the role that each plays in helping your baby to grow stronger every day. There is one other important link in the multidisciplinary chain, however, that was not mentioned. That link is *you*—the parents of the preemie.

At first you might wonder if you should back off and let the doctors and nurses do their jobs. Some parents think, "They know what they're doing, and I don't, so I'll just stay out of the way." But there are a lot of things you can and should do to help the doctors care for your baby. This chapter will discuss some of them. All are medically sound parental involvement activities. Your baby, however, is unique from all other babies. So take a few minutes to check with your pediatrician or neonatologist before you begin.

LEARNING

The first step in parenting a preemie is learning all you can about the baby's state of physical development. During the pregnancy, many parents create a mental picture of how the baby will look when he's born. Your preemie probably looks very different from the way you imagined he would. He looks different from the ones in the full-term baby nursery, and he certainly looks different from the babies in the baby magazines. But in fact, when those babies were at the same age and point of development as your baby is, they looked very much the same; it's just that they were hidden from view inside the uterus. If you want to compare your baby to other babies, get a book that has pictures of the fetus in utero. (*A Child Is Born*, by Lennart Nilsson, Dell Publishing Company, 1986, is a good source.) Then compare your baby to a fetus at the same age of gestation. You'll see that your baby is quite "normal."

Unlike the parents of full-term babies, you have the unique opportunity to actively help your baby grow to "full-term." As you begin to do this, imagine that you're taking a course on premature baby care. As in any other course, it will take time to understand all the facts, but if you read, take notes, and ask questions, you'll soon have all the information you need to love and handle your baby.

Chapters Four, Five, and Six explain the baby's general state of development at the three stages of prematurity. You can get a good start in learning about your baby by carefully reading through the chapter that's appropriate for his weight and age of gestation. Keep in mind while you're reading that not all the information will apply to the individual needs of your baby. As you read, take notes and write down your questions. Then talk to your baby's doctors every day. They're your teachers in this course, and they will have the answers to your questions.

All new parents have a lot to think about. But as the parent of a preemie, you have an additional load of information to process. If you start to feel as if your brain can't hold any more facts, keep in mind that you're not alone. There probably isn't a neonatologist in the world who hasn't answered a late-night phone call to hear, "I know you answered all my questions and explained everything in detail to me this afternoon, but I can't remember what you said. Would you tell me again?" That's why it will be easier to learn about your baby if you get into the habit of writing everything down.

Write down the information you want to remember each day. Record the baby's condition, his medical treatments, his medications, his appearance, his alert periods, and anything else you want to remember. You should also record your own feelings and observations about your baby's growth. Sometimes writing things down on paper and seeing them in black and white can help you view the situation more clearly. It can help you sort your emotional reactions from the actual facts. It will also give you a dated diary that will remind you in the future how far you and your baby have come.

While you're learning about your baby's physical development by reading, taking notes, and asking questions, try to remember the one-day-at-a-time approach to preemie care. Learn all you can about your baby's health today. The doctors can't predict with total accuracy the setback or advance that your baby may encounter tomorrow. Use your time with them to find out about today's developments. Of course, all parents of preemies wonder about tomorrow, and next month, and next year, but it will be easier for you to handle the stress of a premature birth if you make an effort to concentrate on his progress day by day.

As you learn more about your baby each day, you will also have a chance for some hands-on experiences. During the time that your baby was in utero, he was securely cradled, he heard your voice, and he lived with the rhythm and sound of his mother's heartbeat. The environment of the incubator is unfamiliar to the newborn, and the lights and noises of the nursery can be frightening. You are the only source of familiarity your baby has. After birth, you can help give back to him the sense of security that he needs to thrive.

BONDING THROUGH TOUCH

Active parenting usually begins the moment a newborn baby lies in the arms of his mother or father immediately after birth. For the premature baby and his parents, however, that moment may be put off for a few days, or even a few weeks. When a preemie is born and whisked away by a team of doctors and nurses, the parents sometimes feel they've been robbed of a chance to bond with their baby. "I couldn't believe that I wasn't even allowed to hold my own child," said one mother. "Everyone else in the delivery room was looking at her, holding her, and touching her—everyone except me. I had this awful aching need to hold my baby, but the only thing I could do was lie there and cry." It is very difficult to let your baby leave the room when you haven't really had a chance even to meet him, but it should be some comfort to know that the baby is being rushed away to begin the lifesaving medical treatments that are described in Chapter Two. This kind of rapid medical intervention is what will improve your baby's chances of survival so that you will have many opportunities to hold him in the weeks and years to come.

However, you don't have to wait until you can hold your baby in your arms to begin bonding with him. Research now shows that parent-child bonding isn't something that happens only in the first few days after birth. It is a progressive process that develops slowly over a long period of time. You can start this process with your preemie by simply touching him.

All babies need human touch to enhance their mental and physical development, and all parents need to touch their babies to foster emotional attachment. It's the perfect way to establish a warm, positive, parent-child relationship with your preemie even when you can't hold him.

Take a few minutes to prepare yourself each time before you begin. Wash your hands thoroughly for three minutes with soap and water. Make sure your fingernails are cut short. Avoid wearing any jewelry such as bracelets or watches that could scratch the baby's skin, and be sure your hands are warm. It's also better if you don't wear perfume or cologne when your infant is first getting to know you. Let him learn to recognize the natural smell of your skin.

When you first reach through the porthole to touch your baby, take your time. Very slowly and gently rest your hand on his arm or leg. Then with a light featherlike touch, slide your fingers over the surface of his skin.* Start with his arms and legs. Then move to his hands and feet. Watch your child for a response. If this stroking overstimulates your baby, he will show signs of distress, such as a change in color, or in his heart or respiration rate. If that happens, stop the stroking and gently rest your open hand on his back or stomach. If he continues to show distress, stop completely, and try again in a little while. If your baby lies still and seems comfortable with the stroking routine, continue on to his back, shoulders, neck, stomach, face, and head. Always use soft, light strokes and stay alert to signs of discomfort.

---

*Recent literature advocates infant massage for preemies. Be careful how you interpret this advice. The word "massage" implies a technique that involves kneading the muscles beneath the skin. This is not appropriate physical therapy for a small, sick infant.

When your baby is accustomed to the feel of your touch, you can enhance the quality of your time together by also talking to him. Introduce yourself; tell your baby that you love him, and fill him in on all the wonderful things the two of you will do when he comes home. Talk softly because the incubator may magnify and echo the sound of your voice. Then, for as long as he seems to enjoy it, keep touching and talking to let your baby know that you're there.

Soon your baby will be able to come out of the incubator. When he does, you'll be able to further encourage the bonding process by adding holding, cuddling, and kissing to your daily routine. However, at that time, don't stop stroking your baby. Most babies continue to enjoy your stroking and thrive on it long after they come home from the hospital. For many parents it has long-lasting intrinsic benefits. It can give *you* pleasure, confidence, relief from anxiety, a means of communication, and something physical to do for your baby. It can give the *baby* pleasure, comfort, reassurance, a sense of closeness, and emotional and physical contact. That's a lot to gain by simply taking the time to touch.

HOLDING

Exactly when you will hold your baby for the first time depends on his medical needs and his state of development. For the first few weeks it is usually too risky to take smaller premature babies out of their incubators. Besides the problem of disrupting the tubes and wires of the life-support systems, the greatest risk is the danger of exposing them to cold air. This could cause a dangerous dip in body temperature, which would lower the oxygen and glucose levels and raise the metabolic rate.

Most premature babies can be held by their parents, at

least for a few seconds, when their condition is stabilized. This means when they are attached to fewer tubes, when their blood pressure is stable, when they need less supplemental oxygen, and when they no longer have apnea spells during handling. Your baby's doctor is the only one who can tell you exactly when that time will be.

While you're waiting for your baby's condition to stabilize, you may be able to steal a few moments if you pay attention to his daily schedule. Even the very-very premature baby needs to have his diaper changed and to be weighed every day. Ask the nurses when they will be doing these things and try to be there at that time. After you've watched them do it a few times, ask if you can help. This will give you only a few extra minutes of involvement, but while your baby is struggling to grow, every second of physical contact is a bonus for both of you.

Then, when preemies weigh 1500 grams (about three and a quarter to three and a half pounds), are between 32 and 34 weeks postconceptual age, and are medically stable, they are usually able to come out of the incubator for five to ten minutes each day to be held by their parents. The first time this happens is often an emotional and memorable moment. Some parents hold preemies close to their hearts; some hold them at arm's length; some hold on with nervous hands; some hug with confidence. However parents first approach the baby, almost all do it with a pounding heart and teary eyes.

That's not to say that holding your baby will be easy. You shouldn't be disappointed if you don't feel an immediate sense of attachment the moment your arms envelop the baby's tiny frame. Very often it takes time and patience for you to feel comfortable with each other. Sometimes it's difficult to hold preemies because they are still hooked up to intravenous tubes, a cardiac monitor, an oxygen hood, and/or a respirator. The doctor and nurses will be there to help you manage the tubes and wires. After that—relax. Of the eight thousand or so preemies I've worked with, none have suffered any damage because of the way their parents held them. Hold your baby firmly, but without squeezing. You can help him feel secure by holding his arms in close to his body or by swaddling him in a soft blanket. For the time that your baby is in your arms, it doesn't matter how small he is, or how sick he is, or how funny he looks to others; he's yours, and you love him, and nothing else matters.

FEEDING

Providing appropriate and sufficient nourishment is a vital part of your baby's daily care. Because proper nourishment is primary to a baby's growth and development, you baby's doctors will very carefully choose the feeding method that will give him the maximum amount of nutrition and calories. They will make that decision based on his age, medical status, and stability of vital signs. As explained in Chapter Two, at first some babies are fed intravenously with a glucose solution or a total parenteral solution (page 37); others are given oral feedings through an NG tube, which is threaded through the nostrils or mouth down to the stomach (page 42). Some others (especially those 34 weeks gestation or older) are able to bottle- or breast-feed, and many alternate use of the NG tube with bottle- and/or breast-feedings.

Although the doctors will decide which method of feeding is best for your baby, you can still stay actively involved in this vital aspect of his care. First you have to decide if you want to breast- or bottle-feed. This decision isn't a matter of right or wrong; it's a personal choice that you will make based on your own feelings and needs. Some mothers find that breast-feeding has a stabilizing and calming effect on their lives; others find that it adds to the stress of an already difficult time. Some women find breast-feeding easy and trouble-free; others find it laborious and painful. Because parenting a premature baby is in itself a physically and emotionally tiring experience, you have to choose the method of feeding that will make you happy and comfortable. A brief look at both methods follows.

Breast-feeding†

You *can* breast-feed your baby even though he was born prematurely. The exact method of breast-feeding, however, will depend on his age and medical status. A baby born at or after 34 weeks gestation can often be put to the breast shortly after the initial health examination, when all his vital signs are stabilized (which sometimes is on the day of birth). A younger baby who at first is being fed through an NG tube cannot feed directly from his mother's breast. But she can express her milk so that it can be fed to her baby through the tube. When a baby is not yet ready for any kind of oral feeding, his mother can express her milk each day if she wants to maintain the milk flow until the day he is ready. Because of these special circumstances, breast-feeding a premature baby often takes a great deal of time, patience, effort, and persistence. But for many women, it is well worth it.

Some recent medical studies indicate that mothers of premature babies should certainly consider breast-feeding. These studies have found that the mother's milk is tailored to the needs of the preemie. It contains proteins that promote optimal brain growth and development. It has high concentrations of calcium, sodium, and chloride, which are especially needed by preemies. Also, your milk contains a high level of lipase, which is an enzyme that aids in fat

†This section is written specifically to the baby's mother because breast-feeding is primarily her domain.

absorption. (Since preemies need to put on fat, this is an important advantage.) Your milk is desirable because the colostrum (the yellowish fluid secreted from the breasts before the milk comes in) is several times higher in protein than the later milk. This extra protein aids in early body-building and promotes the excretion of bilirubin, which reduces the risk of neonatal jaundice. This colostrum and the later milk are usually absorbed well by the infant and appear to be processed easily by the preemie's immature kidneys. They also pass on to the baby immunity factors that reduce the risk of infections, diarrhea, and perhaps even necrotizing enterocolitis (a serious bowel disease, page 111).

If you decide to breast-feed your premature baby, there is a lot to learn. Older preemies, even if they are immediately ready to suck at the breast, are still not as strong as full-term babies and so their feedings are usually slower and more difficult. Some mothers too quickly give up because they feel, "I just can't do this right." Or, "He won't take enough and I'm afraid he's going to start losing weight." If you really want to breast-feed your child, don't stop when you run into difficulties. Even the mothers of full-term babies often need help, guidance, and support before they and their babies feel comfortable during breast-feedings. Talk to the baby's doctors and nurses, or call a La Leche League member.‡ These people have experience, practical tips, and encouragement to offer.

If your preemie is not yet ready to suck at your breast, you will have to learn how to express your milk and save it for him. The details of how to do this properly cannot be adequately covered in this section on general feeding information. There is so much to say and to explain that whole books have been written on the subject. Some of

‡La Leche League is an international organization dedicated to supporting and encouraging women who want to breast-feed their babies.

these books, along with an informational pamphlet, are listed in Appendix B. Read through these sources, talk to your baby's doctors and nurses, and contact a La Leche League member. They will give you accurate and complete information regarding:

- efficient methods of hand expression
- the benefits and drawbacks of hand-held, battery-operated, and electrical breast pumps
- cleaning and sterilizing your equipment
- when and how to refrigerate or freeze your milk
- how long breast milk will keep
- how to defrost milk safely
- why not to use a microwave
- how to transport milk without spoiling it
- how to promote the let-down reflex without a baby at your breast
- the conditions surrounding the premature birth that may inhibit your milk flow (and how to work around them)
- the kind of diet that will enhance your milk quality and supply.

All of this may sound burdensome at first, but many mothers find that once they get going, it becomes a relaxing and psychologically comforting routine.

If you are undecided about breast-feeding, give it a try. If you start and find it too difficult, you can always switch to formula. At least you'll feel satisfied that you tried, that you gave your baby some of your milk (even the beginning drippings of colostrum are beneficial), and you'll know that in the end you chose what was best for you and for your relationship with your baby.

Jamie didn't know all the details about the medical aspects of breast-feeding her preemie, but she wanted to do it because she needed to be involved in his care. She remembers, "Right after Bobby was born, his doctor asked me if I was going to breast-feed. Since Bobby arrived 9 weeks early, I hadn't really thought about that yet; I didn't know what to say. The doctor told me to think about it and to keep in mind that it would be good for the baby. Since Bobby was being fed through an IV at that time, there was no rush for an answer.

"Later that night I stood to the side of the incubator and watched at least six different people, whom I didn't even know, handle my baby. They poked, pricked, prodded, lifted, turned, diapered, washed, and even kissed this baby who was supposed to be mine. I felt like there was nothing I could do for my own child. That's when I decided to breast-feed. My breast milk was something I could give Bobby that no one else could. By breast-feeding I could take some responsibility for his health. I made the decision very quickly and for very personal reasons, and I stuck by it, but I had no idea at the time how much physical work would be involved.

"Since I knew *nothing* about breast-feeding, I asked one of Bobby's nurses if she could tell me what to do. This nurse was terrific. We sat down and talked for a long time; she gave me some things to read, and she did all she could to encourage and praise my decision. But when we finished, I felt awful. I didn't know that I probably couldn't really breast-feed Bobby for another month. I didn't know I'd have to make time every three or four hours a day and night to express milk so the nurses could put it in little containers attached to the NG tube. I didn't know about the equipment I'd need, and the sterilizing I'd have to do, and the freezing, and storing, and transporting, and on, and on. Just thinking about it made me tired.

"But then I thought about Bobby. I was his mother and I wanted to care for him. I figured that if he had been born at term and had come right home from the hospital, I'd be putting in at least this much time and effort caring for him by myself. That night I called a member of the La Leche

League and I was on my way. She helped me get the breast pump I needed. She came right to my house to show me what to do, and we talked on the phone almost every day for the next two months. Maybe without her constant help, I would have given up (because it's not easy), but now that Bobby is home and breast-feeding with ease, I'm delighted that I didn't quit. Looking back, I think breast-feeding even helped me deal with his prematurity. It gave me something physical to do on a regular schedule that helped keep my baby alive. Of course, the care of the doctors and nurses was vital, but I'm taking some of the credit, too.''

Formula-feeding

Many premature babies are fed with commercial formulas. Like breast-fed babies, they too grow in size and strength. Although breast-feeding can offer the preemie some health benefits that formulas cannot seem to duplicate, there is no research to indicate that in the long-run one fares better than the other. In fact, if you feel strongly about not breast-feeding or find it a painful chore, both you and your baby will be miserable, and that certainly is not what is best.

If you choose to formula-feed, your active involvement in this part of your baby's care will begin when he is ready to start oral feedings. If your baby starts with an NG tube, the doctors will carefully select the formula most appropriate to his needs. It will be introduced gradually in increasing amounts until the doctors are sure the baby's digestive system can tolerate it. (A look into the future shows that soon doctors will be able to type the baby's medical condition into a computer and it will give back the most advantageous feeding formula and schedule.)

If you visit the nursery during feeding time, you can hold the tube as the formula goes into your baby's stomach. The nurses will show you how to hold the tube of formula and how to measure the amount the baby is taking. They will also give you a pacifier to use if the doctors feel sucking during feedings will help your baby's digestive process.

Soon you'll be able to hold your baby in your arms and feed him from a bottle. When you do, remember that feeding is a tiring activity for a preemie. Let him concentrate on sucking. In the beginning, don't try to make eye contact with him, and don't talk or sing to him during feeding time. Find a comfortable place to sit and plan to take your time. Your baby may want to spend more of his feeding time sleeping than eating; the nurses will show you how to gently stimulate him to keep him awake. Try to keep him in a comfortable position that supports his neck and back, and offer him frequent small feedings. Then relax. This is not a race or a contest, and he won't starve while he's learning how to suck on the nipple. If your baby isn't ready to take enough formula by bottle, these feedings will be supplemented with NG tube feedings. Enjoy the opportunity to be together, and give him time to learn how to suck on the nipple.

Liz had planned to breast-feed her second child just as she had her firstborn two years earlier. "Because I had breast-fed Jamie, I knew that breast-feeding was practical, convenient, and emotionally satisfying. It never occurred to me that I would feed formula to my second. But when Kate was born seven weeks early, I quickly changed my mind. I found the whole experience of parenting in the intensive care nursery too physically and mentally draining to add anything else to my daily schedule. The thought of expressing milk every few hours, even though the baby wouldn't use it for quite a while (and then only through a tube!), was more than I could deal with at that time. I thought that I could give the baby more of my time and attention if I conserved my energy. Looking back now, I still think that under different circumstances it would have been nice to have breast-fed Kate, but I don't regret my decision not to. She seemed to thrive on the formula and I don't see any difference now in the health of my two children.''

Like Liz, many mothers decide to formula-feed their premature babies because they need to conserve physical and mental strength. And like Kate, their babies grow into healthy, happy children. If, after you've given breast-feeding serious consideration, you decide to formula-feed your child, be content with that decision and put your energies into other aspects of good parenting.

Whatever the method, your baby's feeding ability will probably become the focus of attention as you patiently wait for him to gain weight and to grow in size and strength. Unfortunately, whether you breast- or formula-feed your baby, he will not keep up the growth rate he would have if he had remained in utero. In the beginning he will lose up to 10 percent of his birth weight; then he will begin to gain weight—but very slowly, because the amount of nourishment and calories he can take in each day is limited by the immature functioning of his digestive system. Of course you want your baby to eat and grow quickly right away, but this is not going to happen. Feeding, like so many other areas of premature baby care, is a slow, one-day-at-a-time process.

BATHING

Preemies are not given "baths" as you probably think of them. Because they must always be protected from drafts and chills, these babies are sponge-bathed every day on the warming table or in their incubator. After you've watched the nurses clean your baby a few times, you can usually take over this daily chore.

Sometimes preemies have negative reactions to soap and lotion, so you will probably wash your baby from head to toe with only warm water and a soft disposable cloth. You will then pat him dry with a soft towel. (All cleaning supplies are kept right in the nursery.)

Most often the baby is washed with his wires and tubes in place. Although you must be very careful not to disturb any IV insertion sites, with practice and care you will soon be able to maneuver your way around them with ease.

After this "bath," you will change the bed linen. Most often this is accomplished without removing the baby from the table or incubator. The nurses will show you how to do it without disturbing the baby or exposing him to drafts.

Just before the baby is ready to go home, the nurses will show you how to bathe him in a small bathtub. By this time his umbilical cord will be healed; he will no longer be attached to tubes and wires; and he will be better able to regulate his body temperature.

DIAPERING

Diapering is one area of preemie care that the nurses will gladly let you do by yourself. The actual diapering technique is exactly the same as it is for a full-term baby: Take off the old diaper; clean the entire diaper area with the cleaning cloths provided in the nursery; and put on the new one (almost all nurseries now use preemie-size disposable diapers).

There are two notable differences in preemie diapering:

1. You must do it while you work around the medical wires and tubes, and while the baby is in the incubator. This does take some practice, but since there is always another diaper to change, eventually you'll get the knack of it.

2. You should never throw away the old diaper. Each diaper is examined for quality and quantity of urine and

feces. When you're finished, just put the dirty diaper aside for the nurse.

You will probably still need preemie-size diapers when you take your baby home. You can use cloth diapers or disposables, but either way you may have to special-order them. (See Appendix B.)

CLOTHING

While your baby is on the warming table or in the incubator, he will not wear much clothing. His skin needs to be fully exposed to the warmed air; so, except for his diaper, he will be naked during most of his stay in the ICN. Even so, some parents enjoy "dressing" their baby in special booties, or hats, or little cotton tops. This is usually fine as long as it doesn't cover the heat sensor probe attached to the baby's skin. That must always be open to the air.

You'll probably find, like most other parents, that your child seems to become more "real-baby-like" as soon as he is in the open bassinet and fully clothed. (Most preemies graduate to bassinets when they are about four pounds.) Clothing seems to give the baby a comfortable, personal, and individualized appearance. Finding clothes that fit, however, is often a difficult task. The very-very and the very premature babies rarely fit into regular newborn clothing sizes, so some parents find doll clothing the most available and most affordable kind of preemie clothing. However, you should keep in mind that doll clothes do not meet any of the government safety or flame-retardant standards. You may also want to make your own clothes, or find stores that stock preemie-size clothing. Most are mail-order catalog stores, however, so it's a good idea to begin looking for preemie clothing while your baby is still in the incubator. (See Appendix B for a partial listing.)

DECORATING AN INCUBATOR

Since the incubator is your baby's first "home," you may want to decorate it in a way that personalizes his environment. Some parents tape fancy name tags or family pictures on the sides. Others decorate with balloons, cartoon characters, and/or festive holiday trimmings. If you also want to give your baby some toys to look at, it's best to buy plastic ones that you can wash thoroughly and then place inside the incubator. Most nurseries have rules against putting stuffed, furry, or cloth toys in the incubator because they attract and hold bacteria. However, if you have such a toy that you really want near the baby, it may be permitted if you put it in a plastic bag.

Mobiles hung outside the incubator may help older babies develop their ability to focus and to interact with the environment. Younger preemies cannot see far enough or focus well enough to enjoy a mobile, but they do seem to enjoy simple black-and-white line drawings. These aren't as decorative as mobiles, but at the younger stages of prematurity they are more practical and helpful.

WHEN ENOUGH IS ENOUGH

In the first week or so after the birth of your child, you may be anxious to spend a great deal of time in the nursery with him. Many parents have said that they couldn't stand the thought of being away from their child at a moment when something went wrong, and so they stayed. But as time passes, and your baby's medical health begins to stabilize, it may not be necessary or desirable to spend every available moment at your baby's side. Especially if your baby will be staying in the hospital for a month or more, you shouldn't feel that you're a "bad" parent if you spend some time doing other things. Many parents feel they're betraying the baby when they have to go back to work; others are torn between spending time with the baby and spending time with their other children. And usually on the bottom of the list is the time allotted for spending with their spouse. At some point, you'll have to decide (without feeling guilty) when enough parenting is enough.

Once your baby's vital signs are stabilized, what he needs most is sleep. Staring at him while he sleeps is not absolutely necessary. If you need to return to work or spend more time at home, do it, and try to arrange a daily visit to the nursery at a time when your baby will be awake or feeding. He still needs to know you're there and he still needs to get to know you. But like any newborn, he does not need every moment of your day.

PARENTING AN ADOPTED OR SURROGATE-CONTRACT PREEMIE

Each state has its own set of laws, rules, and regulations governing adoption and surrogacy. Whatever the specifics in your state, you will not be able to have personal contact with your baby until you have appropriate legal clearance. In some states, this will be within three days after birth, and in others it may not be until thirty days after birth. The baby's health care providers must stick to the letter of the law in these cases to ensure the rights of both the birth mother and the adoptive parents. They can't change the law for you, but talk to the lawyer who is handling the adoption and make sure that you get all the facts about your responsibility, liability, and rights in this kind of special situation.

If you are not able to have immediate, direct contact with the baby, use your waiting time to educate yourself about premature baby care. Read Chapter Two to find out the kinds of routine procedures that are most commonly used in caring for preemies. Also, read the chapter that describes the level of prematurity at which your baby was born. Then get in touch with the social worker at the adoption agency. He or she can give you the support and guidance you'll need during this anxious period.

If you live in a state that allows direct and immediate placement of adopted or surrogate-contract children, then your role in caring for and loving your preemie is no different than that of any other parent. You should visit the baby often; talk to him, touch him, and in every other way possible let him know you're there for him.

Chapter Nine

Going Home

The question asked most frequently by parents of premature babies is "When can my baby come home?" Yet, when that time comes—the time that had been longed for and prayed for—many parents get cold feet. "Already?" they ask. "Don't you think maybe he needs more time to grow?" This is a very natural reaction. The thought of caring for this tiny infant, who has had such close, intensive, personal, round-the-clock care, can be frightening.

The day you take your baby home won't sneak up on you without warning. The attending physicians will talk with you all along about a potential date of discharge. Also, you'll see gradual signs of growth and improvement as, bit by bit, medical equipment is removed. You'll see your baby graduate to breast- or bottle-feedings, and you'll see him progress to a steady weight gain, a stable body temperature, and the ability to breathe independently. If your preemie was originally transferred to a second hospital, you'll watch as he is returned to the hospital of his birth. If he was born in the hospital with an ICN, you'll watch as he is moved to the intermediate care nursery. (The babies in these nurseries are sometimes called "feeders and growers" because, although they no longer need intensive care, they still need the warmth of the incubator and time to grow.) They you'll see your baby grow big enough to come out of the incubator and go into an open bassinet. At that point, you'll know it's almost time to take your baby home.

PREPARING TO GO HOME

There are a number of things to do in the few days before your baby's discharge. If you want your male baby circumcised, now is the time to make those arrangements with the baby's doctors. If you haven't already, now is the time to find a pediatrician who will take primary-care responsibility from the neonatologist when the baby is discharged. You should also contact the hospital social workers at this time. They will be able to help you sort out your financial situation; they can direct you to outpatient services that may be useful to you, and they can give you information about parent support groups that will be of emotional assistance once you're home with the baby. The primary-care nurses will also be able to prepare you for the days at home. They'll show you how to give your baby a tub bath, how to check his temperature, how to suction mucus, and how to know when to call for emergency help. Many nurses also encourage parents to call back to the nursery with any questions or problems that come up once they're home. The neonatologist will talk to you at length about your baby's special needs after discharge. He or she will discuss neonatal follow-up care as well as checkups with specialists if necessary. The developmentalist, for example, may wish to see high-risk babies at regular intervals, sometimes right up to their school years. Also, you will be given explicit instructions regarding feeding schedules, sleep patterns, weight gain, and any necessary medications. Be sure to write everything down because it will be difficult to remember everything once you're home.

If your baby will need complicated care, taking him home can be an unsettling experience. Some hospitals have a special rooming-in arrangement in these circumstances. The night before discharge, the baby and his parents spend the night together in a hospital room. There are no monitors, no nurses, no unrequested assistance. It's a chance for the parents to get comfortable with the idea of "solo" care. If your baby requires specialized care, ask the doctors if your hospital has such a program. If it does, take advantage of the opportunity. It will quickly bring to light any questions or problems that might otherwise not come up until you're home.

Along with these special going-home considerations, of course, there are the traditional preparations. Be sure you have a car seat securely installed to take the baby home. Also, get a full supply of diapers, bottles, nipples, formula, clothing, etc. An ample supply of these everyday necessities is especially vital when bringing home a preemie because, as explained below, it is not a good idea to take a preemie out to the store for the first few weeks. So make sure you have everything you need in advance or have someone on call who can go out to get supplies for you.

AT HOME

Welcome home! You are now about to begin your days as "real" parents. While your baby's doctors and nurses have surely given you instructions specific to your baby's needs, the following sections of this chapter will detail some basics of parenting a preemie at home.

Body Temperature Control

Your baby is now able to self-regulate his body temperature, but he probably still lacks the full degree of body fat necessary to brave the elements. Therefore, although you don't have to turn up the heat to an uncomfortable level, use the following guidelines to keep your baby comfortable whether indoors or out:

Air Temperature	*Clothing Needs*
over 80°	a T-shirt and diaper
between 75° and 80°	one more layer of clothing than you wear
between 70° and 75°	two more layers of clothing than you wear
below 70°	two more layers of clothing than you wear, *plus* a blanket and a hat

If your baby has had body temperature control problems in the nursery, be sure to ask if you should take any other special precautions against exposure.

Infection Control

A preemie's immune system is still quite immature; this makes him especially vulnerable to colds and other communicable diseases. However, if the weather is nice and you dress your baby appropriately (see "Body Temperature Control"), you certainly can take him outside for fresh air without risking illness. If you're careful not to expose him to direct sunlight or drafts, he'll probably benefit from a carriage ride around the block or to the park. But do *not* take him to crowded indoor places such as a shopping mall. Your pediatrician can best advise you how long you should keep your baby out of crowds, but six weeks is usually recommended.

To avoid spreading infections, it is a very wise health practice to continue the precautions you always took when you visited your baby in the nursery. In the beginning, limit the amount of company you welcome into your home. Then ask the guests who do visit to wash their hands before touching the baby, and suggest that they don't hold the baby close to their clothing. Also, make sure that you, your spouse, and your other children wash your hands frequently. In time your child will develop the antibodies he needs to combat infection, but for the first month or so at home, you can safeguard his health by taking these few precautions.

In your efforts to safeguard your child's health, it is also vital to ban cigarette smoking in your house. Allowing your preemie to be a "passive smoker" exposes him to an irritant that can interfere with his oxygenation, cause him to wheeze, and make him more susceptible to pneumonia and respiratory tract infections. Passive smoking is bad for all children, but for your preemie it is an especially dangerous toxin. If you smoke, quit, or go outside when you smoke. If your guests smoke, explain your baby's health condition and insist that they don't smoke in your home. If you want, put No Smoking signs around your house. Do whatever you have to do to give your baby clean air to breathe.

Feeding

Even now that you're home, feeding times may still be the focal point of each day. Before you leave the hospital, your baby's doctors will give you very specific information about feeding methods and schedules, but if you had the opportunity to feed your baby while he was in the hospital, you will feel quite comfortable doing it now. Your baby will probably still feed very frequently (about every three hours). He will also continue to feed slowly until he grows stronger and more proficient at coordinating his sucking, swallowing, and breathing.

If your baby is being bottle-fed, he may have grown accustomed to the red preemie nipples used in the nursery. These nipples allow more fluid to flow through with less sucking. You probably have brought a few home with you, but now it's time to slowly introduce regular nipples that will help your baby develop a stronger suck.

If you are breast-feeding, you may still find it necessary to give some of the feedings by bottle. At discharge, most preemies still do not have the physical strength to breast-feed seven or eight times each day. Most can feed at the breast once or twice, and take the bottle (which allows the milk to flow easily) for the other feedings. You will probably continue to express and store milk for these bottle-feedings at least until the baby has reached "full-term." By that time all the days of pumping and storing may be behind you, and your baby will be at your breast for every feeding. Like bottle-fed babies, breast-fed babies too may still feed frequently and slowly, so continue to be patient. Now that you no longer have the guidance and support of the nurses, you may want to contact a La Leche League member (the number is in the white pages of the phone book), who can offer the encouragement you may need to keep going.

Sleeping

Your baby will still do more sleeping than anything else because he still has a lot of catch-up growing to do. When you bring him home keep in mind the kind of sleeping environment he is used to. Obviously, he does not need a quiet, darkened room to sleep; in fact, this environment may scare him. At first, let him sleep with the light and radio on. Gradually reduce the bulb wattage down to a night-light, and the radio down to a soft hum.

Many parents worry about putting a preemie to sleep in his own bedroom. They worry that he may stop breathing or may need them but won't be able to cry out for help. To ease the stress of this concern, preemies are best kept in a small portable cradle or bassinet. During the day, you can keep your baby close by in the living room or kitchen. At night you can keep him next to your own bed, where you can easily check him and feed him. Some parents sleep in the baby's room so they can keep a close watch, but this certainly isn't best for their own sleep needs (or for the marriage). It is *never* a good idea to bring your baby into your own bed.

Your baby needs his sleep and so do you. Take advantage of the times your baby sleeps to get rest for yourself. Staying up to stare at your child while he sleeps won't make him grow stronger or healthier; it will only make you more tired. The doctors would not have discharged your infant if he still needed round-the-clock observation. Your baby has grown and matured to the point where he can regulate his own breathing (unless he is at home on respiratory monitors or equipment), and that's why he's at home with you. It's time to relax, settle into a manageable routine, and enjoy your baby.

Behavior

Premature infants tend to have slightly different behavior patterns than full-term babies. As a group, they tend to be more irritable and less easily consoled. This fussiness will subside as the body systems (especially the central nervous system) mature, but until then there are a number of soothing techniques you can use to comfort your baby.

Your preemie may not have a loud lusty cry, so he will express his discomfort through other physical signs such as a change in skin color, repeated yawning or hiccupping, flailing arms and legs, or general crankiness. When he does this, you can give him a sense of security by holding and/or swaddling him in a receiving blanket. When you hold your baby, bring his arms and legs into his body so he is in the fetal position; this will make him feel more comfortable and help him develop flexion. Don't worry that you'll spoil your baby by holding him too much. Until he is at least three months corrected age your baby needs to be held as often as you can make time to do it. When you swaddle your infant, be sure to pull his arms in across his chest and wrap him securely. Many parents soothe their baby by putting him in a body sling or carrier. This way the baby is held close to the parent; he feels the warmth of the body and hears the beating of the heart, and the parent has both hands free to do other things.

Some babies are soothed with a pacifier. If your baby doesn't want the new one you offer him, it may be because he's accustomed to the one the nurses gave him in the hospital. Probably this was just a nipple off a preemie bottle. Try it. Take a bottle nipple; stuff it with gauze and tape over the open bottle end. This will prevent the baby from sucking in air, and it will give him the kind of pacifier he is comfortable with.

Sucking is very soothing for a baby, so he may quiet down if you offer him food, but this isn't a good habit to get into. If your baby cries when it's not his feeding time, try other methods of soothing before you give him food. Even preemies can be overfed and can be taught to think of food as comfort rather than nourishment. It's best to keep your baby well fed on schedule and find other ways to comfort him between feedings.

In addition to these periods of irritability, you many worry that something is wrong with your baby when he doesn't respond to stimuli such as your smile, your voice, or tickling. It is a wonderful feeling when infants begin to interact by smiling or cooing, but your preemie may not be developmentally ready to do that yet. Even when he passes his due date and is considered "full-term," he has a lot of catching up to do. If your baby shows no response to any stimuli, call your pediatrician and tell him about it. But most often parents of preemies have to wait just a little longer before they see that joyful show of delight from their baby.

As you watch your baby for signs of behavioral development, *always* use your baby's corrected age to judge his abilities. This corrected age is calculated by adding the chronological age to the number of weeks he was born prematurely. For example, Karin was born 8 weeks (2 months) early; therefore, when she is four months old, her corrected age will be two months. When you read books that say, for example, that your child should roll over at four months of age, remember that for your child, that expectation is only valid at his *corrected* age.

The corrected-age concept makes perfect sense in terms of physical and developmental expectations. It is a bit confusing, however, to people who have no understanding of prematurity. Many parents of preemies find themselves fumbling through the full explanation of prematurity, and chronological age vs. corrected age when a stranger in the supermarket says, "What a cute baby. How old is she?" Save yourself time and trouble by answering immediately with the corrected age. In later life, those few weeks or months between birth date and due date will mean nothing, but in infancy they can make a big difference in a baby's appearance and abilities.

Family Relationships

Now that your preemie is home, you can begin to put all your other family relationships back in order. The siblings who felt ignored while you spent time in the nursery will need more of your attention to reassure them of your love. If it is at all possible, ask a trusted sitter to watch the preemie occasionally while you take your other child out, away from the baby. At least once a day find a small space of time that is only for the two of you. Both of you will still have adjustments to make, but this special time together will let a sibling know that his or her life is also of great value to you.

Now that the baby is home, you may finally have time to get to know your spouse again. The two of you have been through a lot during the baby's time in the hospital. Some couples find that the experience brings them closer together; others find that it fosters emotional and sexual incompatibilities. Whatever the state of your marital relationship, take time for each other. Now that your baby is well on his way to good health, make every effort to get out of the house *alone.* Go out for dinner, or a game of tennis, or even just a long walk. Your preemie will still demand a great deal of your time and attention, but he will also benefit from a happy family environment.

It sounds like a tall order to (1) take care of your preemie, (2) take care of your other children, (3) take care of your spouse, and (4) take care of yourself. But what it comes down to is a normal family life that does not continually cater to the needs of one at the expense of the others.

Special Circumstances

Quite frequently preemies are sent home while still on apnea monitors or respiratory support systems. This growing
trend allows babies who are otherwise ready to go home
the chance to cut down on the length of their hospital stay.
This is desirable because the home environment can enhance the baby's neurological and emotional development,
and also, of course, because it is a much less expensive way
to give the baby the care he needs.

The care of babies on home-care equipment can be quite
involved and is therefore closely supervised by doctors,
respiratory therapists, and, usually, visiting nurses, who will
stay between four and twenty-four hours a day depending
on the need. "David's Story" on page 166 will give you a
glimpse of what it's like to care for an oxygen-dependent
child at home, but the full details of home respiratory management are far too complex and extensive to be covered
adequately in this book. If your baby comes home with
respiratory support equipment, the doctors, nurses, and
therapists will very carefully instruct and train you in how
to use it. Although such care is time-consuming and complex, parents eventually learn how to manage the systems
in much the same way that other parents learn how to diaper and bathe their babies—out of necessity and with
practice.

Babies who are severely handicapped will also need special home-care management. Again, this care can be very
involved and highly specialized, but the neonatologist, pediatrician, neurologist, pediatric developmentalist, and
physical therapists will keep in close touch with the parents
to guide and support them as they learn how to care for
the special needs of their baby.

Whether your baby comes home at four pounds or at
seven, whether he is breathing independently or is depen-

dent on machines, whether he is developmentally normal or handicapped, what he needs most is your time, your attention, and your love. Preemies have a special claim on all the good things in life because they worked so hard to survive and enjoy it. You too have earned the right to relax and enjoy this child who came into the world a bit early, but who is now here to stay.

Chapter Ten

Paying for a Preemie

O f all the questions you'll ask about your baby's medical care, "How much does it cost?" is one that probably will never cross your lips. Like all parents, you want the best possible care for your child no matter what the cost, because there is no price tag that can be placed on the value of your child's life.

Information about paying for a preemie is included in this book precisely because it *is* the last thing on your mind. Before the birth of your baby, you may have been financially astute and organized, but now, when health and emotional issues are foremost in your thoughts, money matters may be ignored, and then, when they can no longer be ignored, they may already have become overwhelming. Let this chapter guide you step-by-step through the money management aspects of parenting a preemie. It's understandable why you might say, "I don't care about the money!" But if, for example, your insurance company refuses to pay for any of your baby's care because you never called to add him to your policy, you will care. Keep in mind as you read this chapter that the total cost, as well as the billing and payment procedures, vary from state to state, and with each hospital, doctor, and insurance company. The following information is presented as a general overview of the basics.

FOR PARENTS WITH INSURANCE COVERAGE

It's not unusual for parents to feel secure simply because they have "health insurance." It's also not unusual for the health insurance coverage to be inadequate for intensive neonatal care. Some policies cover the hospital bills, but not the doctor bills. Some cover a healthy newborn, but not complicated neonatal care. Some automatically cover the newborn; others will not cover the baby until they are notified of the birth.

The only way to be absolutely sure of which expenses your insurance policy does or does not cover is to call your personnel officer if you have group insurance, or the insurance company representative if you have an individual policy. It is best if you call while you're still pregnant to tell the representative that, when your baby is born, you want him added to your policy. If this is not done in advance of the birth, you may have to call the day the child is born to be completely covered. A parent who calls the insurance representative four days after the birth may be told that any expenses incurred during those first four days are not covered. You also should definitely call your insurance representative to notify him of a multiple birth; sometimes, insurance companies reject bills for multiple births because they think they are duplicates. You can avoid confusion and delays be letting your insurance company representatives know you've had a baby, the status of his condition, and the expected length of his hospital stay.

Billing and Payment

Sometimes the hospital and/or doctor will send your bills directly to the insurance company. Some companies pay the doctor directly; others will send the payment to you. Other times the hospital and/or doctor will send the bills to you, and you will submit them to the insurance company. How do you know what to do? Ask. Find out exactly what kind of insurance coverage you have and how the payment of bills will be handled by each doctor. Call your baby's doctors and your insurance company representative and ask them the questions on the checklist below.

Questions to Ask Your Insurance Company Representative

Is my policy or my spouse's the primary carrier?
Are hospital bills covered?
Are doctor bills covered?
Is my baby covered for extended neonatal care?
Is there a deductible amount that I must first pay?
   If yes, what is that amount?
What percentage of the bills will you pay?
Is there a limit to my policy coverage?
   If yes, what is that limit?
Is there a point at which you will begin to pay 100 percent of the bill?
   If yes, at what point will that happen?
Will you make payment to me or the health care provider?
Will you pay miscellaneous expenses such as transportation to the hospital, hotel stays near the hospital, a breast pump, home-care monitoring equipment, visiting and skilled nursing service?

Questions to Ask Your Baby's Doctors

Do you have my insurance policy information?
Are you a participating doctor in my insurance company?
Will you bill me or the insurance company?

Once you have these answers, set up a payment system that you can begin to follow as soon as the bills start to arrive. If you shove all bills, paid and unpaid, into a drawer for the first three months, you may be adding to the strain of parenting a preemie. You might want to try this method of payment:

Step One

Divide your bills into these four categories:
1. mother's hospital bills
2. mother's doctor bills
3. baby's hospital bills
4. baby's doctor bills

Step Two

Find out from your employer or insurance company representative who has the primary insurance coverage for each of the four categories listed above. Most often, if the baby's mother and father both have insurance coverage, the mother's insurance company is the primary carrier for her own bills and the father's insurance company provides secondary coverage for her bills. This means that the mother's bills should first be submitted to her insurance company and the balance of what that company doesn't pay can be sent to the father's insurance company. On the other hand, the father's insurance company is usually the primary carrier for the baby's bills, while the mother's insurance company is the secondary carrier. (This holds true even if the mother and father are not married but the father claims paternity.)

Step Three

Pay all bills up to your deductible amount.

Step Four

Submit all medical bills to your insurance company. Be sure to clarify whether the payments should be sent to you or to the health care provider. Most companies pay 80 percent of medical costs.

Step Five

Find out which doctors involved in your child's care are participating members in your insurance company's program. Participating doctors must accept the insurance company's payment as full payment and cannot pass any remaining balance on to you. This is important for you to know. If you are mistakenly billed by one of the participating doctors for a balance, you should write a note on the bill stating that because he or she is a participating doctor, the insurance company's remittance is considered full payment.

Step Six

If the doctor is not a participating member in your insurance company, send the remainder of the bill to your spouse's insurance company. If your doctor is not participating, and your spouse does not have insurance coverage, you are responsible for the remaining bill.

Step Seven

Make sure the insurance company makes their payment on the full amount submitted. Sometimes an insurance company will pay on an amount that is less that the doctor's fee. If, for example, you submit a bill for $400, the insurance company may respond with payment on only $275, which they claim is the appropriate fee for the stated care. If this happens, call the doctor's office, explain the situation, and ask the doctor to write a letter to the insurance company justifying his fee. Very often the insurance company has paid the going rate for routine child or adult care without realizing that the procedure involved specialized neonatal care and physicians. This additional information often enables the insurance company to readjust the claim and pay on the full amount submitted.

FOR PARENTS WITHOUT INSURANCE COVERAGE

If you do not have health insurance, the hospital's social worker will help you find social service agencies that can give you financial aid. For example, he or she will determine if you are eligible for Medicaid insurance. Eligibility for this federal program, which is state-administered and county-run, is based on income, assets, and family size. The social worker may also contact your county Board of Social Services to help you apply for financial assistance from Aid to Families with Dependent Children (AFDC) and/or Women, Infants, and Children (WIC) funds.

When your baby is ready to come home, a social-service case manager will help you find the resources you'll need for home care. For example, you may be able to receive home energy assistance from the county to help you heat your home to the temperature your baby needs. You may also be eligible for food stamps, and organizations like the Easter Seal Society may even pay for phone installation so you can maintain ongoing contact with your baby's health care providers.

You may have planned and saved to pay for the birth of your baby, but now that you have to provide for the special needs of a premature infant, which can cost up to $300,000, let the social worker help you find the financial assistance you'll need.

OTHER SOURCES OF FINANCIAL ASSISTANCE

Whether you have health insurance or not, look to local agencies and organizations for additional help in meeting the cost of caring for your baby. You may be able to get financial aid for costs not covered by Medicaid or your own insurance company. Start this search by contacting the hospital's social service department; a social service worker will help you determine where you can best find financial aid. If you expect your baby to be in the hospital for more than thirty days, for example, you may automatically qualify for institutional Medicaid insurance. Also, every state has a child health service agency (sometimes called Crippled Children's Program or Special Child Health Services) that, depending on the baby's diagnosis, may be able to offer financial assistance. And families who have catastrophic health-care bills may also be eligible for federal aid programs. Ask the social worker at your baby's hospital for this information.

In addition to government-subsidized programs, you may be able to get help from private organizations. The cost of home-care equipment, visiting nurse service, travel to and from the hospital, hotel stays (if your baby is transferred to a hospital far away), babysitters for siblings, a breast pump, psychological counseling, etc., is occasionally covered by insurance if your doctor writes a prescription or note of explanation, but most often these are out-of-pocket expenses.

With the help of the social worker, contact the United Way, which can refer you to agencies and organizations that may be able to help you. The Easter Seal Society also gives referrals, as well as providing a limited home-equipment loan service. La Leche League may be able to supply a breast pump if you need one, and the Red Cross sometimes can help with transportation problems and may sponsor a parent support group that can give you emotional care. Hometown groups such as the Elks, Rotary, Women's Club, Shriners, and those that are church-affiliated may also lend a hand if you ask.

Parenting a premature baby can drain your attention and energy, as well as your financial resources. Seek out those who can help you and accept assistance when it's available. This is one more way to make this difficult time a bit easier.

Chapter Eleven

. . . .

A Question of Ethics

This book has highlighted many of the medical advances made in neonatology over the last ten years that have given your premature baby an optimal chance of survival. Aggressive neonatal care, which includes delivery room resuscitation, heart and respiratory monitoring, assisted respiration, and varied means of nutrition delivery, has improved the survival rate of all babies born prematurely. However, as these technological advancements allow physicians to improve the survival rates of increasingly smaller preemies, ethical questions often arise. At this point, no one has exact answers to these questions. This chapter strives merely to acknowledge their existence, state the facts as they are known today, and share the ethical dilemmas faced by some parents of preemies.

• **Question 1**: As increasing numbers of smaller and less mature preemies survive, aren't we also increasing the numbers of severely handicapped children who come into the world?

It's true that the tinier the baby, the more likely he is to have long-term neurological, developmental, physical, and/or intellectual handicaps, because these babies are more prone to seizures, grade 4 hemorrhage, and infection. However, compared to the relative number of very-very low-birth-weight babies who survive without any kind of handicaps, the number of handicapped infants graduating from intensive care nurseries is still much smaller than it was in 1960.

The graph below shows the outcome of 1,000 very-low-birth-weight babies (those less than 1500 grams or about 3 pounds 5 ounces). The number of developmentally normal babies who survived in this 1960 study was a mere 72 out of 1,000; while 67 survived with severe handicaps—a number almost equal to the number of developmentally normal. In 1985 the number of developmentally normal children jumped to 568 out of 1,000; while 101 had severe handicaps—only one-fifth the number of the developmentally normal. These numbers clearly show that modern medicine is increasing the survival rate of well babies in much greater proportion than handicapped ones.

However, these statistics may mean very little to parents like Joan and Craig whose daughter, Faith, was born at 25 weeks gestation weighing 600 grams (about 1 pound 5 ounces). Faith is now one year old and severely handicapped. She suffers varying degrees of speech, vision, and hearing impairment; she has weekly physical therapy sessions to help her compensate for her lack of large and small motor skills, and her I.Q. is below 70. "When Faith was first born," Joan recalls, "we wanted the doctors to do whatever they could to save her life. And they did. But now we look at the quality of her life and wonder if it wouldn't have been better if she were born twenty years ago when she would have been left to die a natural death."

For parents like Joan and Craig, for all the health care

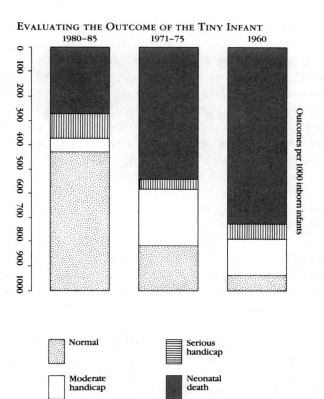

Outcomes of extremely low birthweight infants (≤ 1000 gm) born in level III hospitals from 1960 to 1985. From U.S. Congress, Office of Technology Assessment, *Health Technology Case Study 38: Neonatal Intensive Care for Low Birthweight Infants: Costs and Effectiveness* (Washington, D.C.: United States Government Printing Office, December 1987). Used with permission.

providers involved in the care of handicapped preemies, and for the society in which they live, there is always the nagging question, "Was it right to save these babies?" No one has the "right" answer.

• **Question 2:** Where is the line between too immature to live and mature enough to survive?

In 1976 the World Health Organization defined fetuses weighing less than 500 grams (about 1 pound 2 ounces) as incapable of sustaining life. In the United States the definition varies from state to state, with some defining "viable" as any newborn showing signs of life. However, with the current methods of care, most medical professionals feel that the biological line of survival outside the uterus is drawn at 23 to 24 weeks gestation, or at a weight of between 500 to 600 grams (about 1 pound 2 ounces to 1 pound 6 ounces), even though very few (less than 10 percent) born at this weight or gestation will survive.

The ethical conflict in this low-age viability line lies in the allowable age for legal abortions. It seems that medicine may have outpaced law in this area. In a 1979 decision in the case of *Colautti v. Franklin*, the Supreme Court ruled that the exact moment of viability for an infant cannot be determined by law, but must be left to the judgment of the attending physician. Therefore, it is certainly possible for a woman to be in one of the hospital's operating rooms for an abortion of her 24-week old-fetus, while in the next room, doctors are striving to sustain the life of an infant born prematurely at 24 weeks gestation.

Fran's baby, for example, was born at 24 weeks gestation weighing just over 1 pound. "The doctors tell us that our baby may experience some neurological and development problems as she grows, and may even be learning impaired," says Fran. "But we call him a miracle and we are very grateful to all the doctors, nurses, and everybody else who worked hard to keep him alive." Saving a 24-week-old preemie does not cause any ethical problems for parents such as Fran.

On the other hand, Sheri doesn't feel the same about her baby and the doctors who kept him alive. "I went into the hospital for an abortion," she says. "It was a very difficult decision for me to make. (I guess that's why I waited so long.) But I finally realized that I could not give this child the life he deserved. I'm not emotionally, financially, or mentally ready for a baby. My obstetrician said it was not too late to abort at 24 weeks. After the procedure, thinking the decision and the abortion were behind me, I found out that the baby was resuscitated in the delivery room. What was supposed to be an aborted fetus is now a neurologically impaired infant. I don't think it's right that these doctors give life to a baby too small to develop normally and then send him packing with a parent who can't take care of him properly. It's just not right." Parents like Sheri sometimes feel that both law and medicine have let them down.

The questions of what's right or wrong, and what's too small or not too small are impossible to answer with absolutes. Each premature birth presents a unique set of circumstances that has to be evaluated on an individual basis. In the field of neonatology, very often one answer only leads to another question.

• **Question 3:** Is it right to continue aggressive treatment for infants who may not have much of a chance for survival?

In this question, the conflict lies in the phrase, "*much* of a chance." Neonatologists can initially try to judge a preemie's chances of survival based on his birth age and weight. They can extend their prediction based on his response to delivery room resuscitation and his Apgar scores. But then comes the fuzzy area where, based on past experiences, physicians must try to determine the final outcome for the baby if aggressive treatment is continued, as well as if aggressive treatment is discontinued. Sometimes the baby's medical status is clearly deteriorating (because, for example, he is comatose or has a massive grade 4 hemorrhage), and therefore the doctors can predict with certainty that the baby will be severely handicapped or will die shortly. In these cases aggressive treatment may not be continued. (Legally, care is not required for those infants for whom the care is "virtually futile," and those for whom dying would merely be prolonged.) But when a baby has "some" chance of survival and the long-term outcome is not so clearly predictable, physicians face a much more difficult decision about whether or not to continue aggressive care.

The Abotts don't feel that the doctors should have worked so aggressively to keep their very sick preemie alive. "I don't know if she felt the pain of all the procedures, tests, and monitoring she was subjected to," says the baby's dad, "but I can't imagine that she was able to enjoy even one moment of her life. Since it seemed obvious from the beginning that she was going to die, they should have left her alone to die in peace and with dignity. Now all I have are painful memories and two hundred thousand dollars in bills for a baby who is dead."

On the other hand, more and more frequently there are stories of premature babies who beat the odds—who survive even though their parents were told to begin making funeral arrangements. Should extensive support be withheld from all very sick preemies even though some could survive to live quality lives? What guidelines can be "correct" when, for example, in 1988 an Oakland, California, preemie was born weighing only 440 grams (about 15 ounces) and went home to her family weighing 4 pounds 10 ounces? Then again in 1989 a Camden, New Jersey, preemie was born weighing only 15 ounces, and the doctors gave her less than a 5 percent chance of survival. But after five months of aggressive treatment, Chrissy's survival was heralded in a news headline that read, "Miracle baby beats odds and goes home."

Life-and-death decisions are always difficult and sometimes painful to make. If past medical experiences say a child has a "slim" chance of survival, should parents and doctors offer aggressive treatment in the hope that this is one who will make it? There is no easy answer.

• **Question 4**: Who should decide whether or not to continue aggressive treatment?

There is no ethical conflict involved when aggressive treatment enables a child to grow to be perfectly normal and healthy. In these cases the parents, the doctors, the law, and society encourage continued supportive care. However, when there is a quality-of-life question involved (which is measured by the likelihood of handicap or impairment), the determination of who should be allowed to "pull the plug" can become a legal and ethical dilemma.

The physician's role in determining the continuance of supportive treatment for most preemies has been federally regulated by the *Baby Doe* case of 1982. Baby Doe was born with Down's Syndrome and an interrupted esophagus which prevented him from swallowing any food. The baby's physicians and family chose not to treat the esophagus problem (which might have been surgically corrected) because of the Down's Syndrome condition. The baby died before the family's right to withhold treatment was ruled on in a court of law. However, one month after the death of Baby Doe in Bloomington, Indiana, the U.S. Department of Health and Human Services issued what is called "Notice to Health Care Providers." This notice informed hospital administrators and doctors that they risk losing federal funding if they withhold medically indicated treatment or nourishment from handicapped newborns. In 1985 the regulation was further expanded to define "withholding medically indicated treatment" as

the failure to respond to the infant's life-threatening conditions by providing treatment (including appropriate nutrition, hydration, and medication), which, in the treating physician's (or physicians') reasonable medical judgement, will be most likely to be effective in ameliorating or correcting all such conditions. . . .

Three separate exceptions to the rules are:

1. The infant is chronically and irreversibly comatose;
2. The provision of such treatment would merely prolong dying, not be effective in ameliorating or correcting all of the infant's life-threatening conditions, or otherwise be futile in terms of the survival of the infant; or
3. The provision of such treatment would be virtually futile in terms of the survival of the infant, and the treatment itself under such circumstances would be inhumane.

The phrase in this regulation that still leaves the decision to discontinue support open to debate is: "reasonable medical judgement." In an effort to create institutional guidelines that would establish what exactly this is, many hospitals have now formed Infant Care Review Committees—often called Infant Bioethics Committees. These committees are comprised of hospital administrators, attending physicians, various medical specialists, and the families involved in each individual case. As a group, they can evaluate the case, judge the probable outcome of continued care, and inform each other of any extenuating circumstances. They also formulate guidelines for physicians and families and offer support and educational information.

The family's input is vital to the existence of these committees. The parents are ultimately the child's primary care-givers and they are better informed than anyone else regarding the nonmedical aspects of the baby's future. Their wishes concerning the continuance or removal of life-supporting treatments should be seriously considered when determining the future course of action. In fact, a President's Commission has recommended that situations of unmanageable ethical ambiguity regarding newborn care be resolved by following the parents' wishes.[1]

The decision to continue or to stop medical treatment for your baby should not be made quickly or rashly. It should be made in conference with your baby's doctors. Talk to them. Ask their opinions. Encourage them to be open and honest with you so that you can make an informed yet compassionate decision regarding the extent of supportive care you want for your baby.

In answer to the question, "Who has the last word?" the answer (as with most ethical issues) is: "It depends."

A case in point was recently presented in *Clinics in Perinatology*.[2] The case involved a five-day-old infant with severe birth defects. During treatment the child went into cardiac arrest and required closed-chest resuscitation. After thirty minutes he was pronounced dead by the pediatric cardiologist. Within seconds after leaving the room, the physician was called back because the infant's heart had resumed beating. The baby was put on a respirator and sent to the intensive care nursery. After hearing what had happened, and after many days of testing, the parents asked that respiratory assistance be discontinued. The attending physician did not want to do this and he requested that the pediatric ethics committee consider the case. At the committee meeting, a pediatric neurologist indicated that because the child had a nearly flat EEG test result, lacked response to pain or stimulation, and was not able to breathe spontaneously, it was highly unlikely that the child would ever recover cognitive function. Because the child had apparently suffered neurologic devastation, it was no longer

1. The President's Commission for the Study of Ethical Problems in Medicine and Biomedical and Behavioral Research, *Deciding to Forego Life-sustaining Treatment* (Washington, D.C.: United States Government Printing Office, March 1983).
2. Mary B. Mahowald, "Baby Doe Committees: A Critical Evaluation," *Clinics in Perinatology* 15, no. 4:789–800. (1988)

clear that his interests were best served by continuing respiratory support. Committee members agreed that it was appropriate to discontinue treatment. The attending physician, however, still felt morally uneasy about discontinuing respiratory support, and so at the committee's recommendation, he transferred care to another doctor. Within a few days, respiratory support was withdrawn, and the infant died.

In this case the review committee agreed with the parents' wishes to discontinue life-support systems rather than with the physician's feelings of moral obligation. In other cases, review committees might decide against the parents' requests. In any case, the best outcome for the child is attained through the joint efforts of parents and physicians who sit down together and talk about the facts, the future outlook, and their feelings. In the vast majority of cases this kind of face-to-face discussion leads to a mutually satifying decision.

· **Question 5**: Medical technology is allowing smaller preemies to survive, but at what cost?

In 1988 an article in *Newsweek* magazine estimated the cost of four months' intensive neonatal care to be $366,480.[3] Keeping this cost in mind, a 1989 *New York Times* article asked its readers to consider the cost of caring for low-birth-weight babies who are born to drug-abusing mothers who may abandon them or lose custody of them. The article went on say that these babies are overwhelming the public hospital system in New York City and challenging the city's social services and adoption agencies. It stated in reference to these preemies, "They are both a medical

3. Barbara Kantrowitz et al., "Preemies," *Newsweek*, 16 May 1988, 62–67.

miracle and a public health problem.''[4] Viewed in this light the "cost" of a preemie goes far beyond the dollar amount stated on a hospital bill. Society as a whole pays a price for intensive neonatal care. Our health insurance premiums may reflect the increasing number of premature births; our taxes respond to the increased demands on government-funded programs such as Medicaid; our hospital bills are adjusted to accommodate the indigent and uninsured; our state and local social service agencies and the public educational systems that work with the handicapped and learning disabled are supported by all of us.

However, when adding up these figures, it's important to remember that they are compounded by the same chain reaction involved in the technological advancements that now extend the lives (as well as the hospital stay) of many neurologically, developmentally, and/or physically disabled full-term infants, as well as cancer and cardiac patients, transplant recipients, and accident victims. No one would suggest that these patients be denied care because the cost might trickle down to the community. It's apparent that looking only at the financial cost of medical care is short-sighted. It's important to remember that the vast majority of premature babies grow to be healthy, contributing members of society. (Consider, for example, Isaac Newton, Mark Twain, Winston Churchill, Pierre Auguste Renoir, Anna Pavlova, and Sidney Poitier, who were all born prematurely.) To consider, for the sake of fiscal savings, withholding aggressive treatment for all preemies whose medical outlook cannot be determined as perfect at the moment of birth is a graphic example of throwing the baby out with the bathwater.

Human life has a value far too high for a price tag. But

4. Howard W. French, "Tiny Miracles Become Huge Public Health Problem," *New York Times*, 19 February 1989, sec. 1, 44.

the cost of preserving life can be very high. The answer to the question of who pays the emotional and financial price for intensive neonatal care is, of course: first, the parents, and then the community as a whole. But then the answer to the question of who benefits from intensive neonatal care is also: first, the family, and then the community as a whole.

Ethical issues and neonatal care have come to be closely associated. It is often difficult to separate them, but it is also difficult to address them properly because all the facts are not yet in. Because most of the technological advancements that prompt these questions have been made only in the last ten years, there are few studies of the long-term effects of the "new" methods of intervention. Also, researchers are now making discoveries about the role of genetics, chromosomal abnormalities, and brain functioning, for example, that may make older studies invalid. If it is true (as some studies now indicate) that cerebral palsy, for example, is not related to any definable birth defect, but is rather related to inherited or prenatal factors, then all the statistics that include cerebral palsy as a handicap of prematurity must be reevaluated.

The adage that says, "The more we learn, the less we know," is certainly true when discussing ethical issues. In the face of quality-of-life questions, I have found that many people in the field of neonatology are becoming increasingly concerned over the fate of their patients, the direction of their actions, and the meaning of their work. As a group, neonatologists tend to believe that all babies born alive deserve a chance at survival. In the delivery room they will resuscitate a newborn who is having difficulty breathing and, if he responds well to this resuscitation, in most cases aggressive medical treatment is warranted.

In those few moments after birth when these decisions are made, it is impossible to know which babies will have handicaps, which will be normal, or even which will survive. Modern medicine simply can't guarantee perfection, but we can guarantee that all babies (even when it's apparent they will die) are kept as pain-free and as comfortable as possible. Even with all the advances made in the last few years, some preemies will still die. Some die despite our efforts; some die because of our efforts (yes, even in neonatology there is room for human error)—but everyone involved in the care of these babies does his or her best. Today, the overwhelming odds are in favor of the baby's survival and of his living a normal life.

As the field of neonatology continues to explore life and expand its capabilities, we will surely find that the ethical questions posed in this chapter are only the tip of a mammoth iceberg. As new issues arise, the fields of medicine, law, and social services, as well as the community, will need to continue to join forces and together decide what is "right" and what is "wrong."

Epilogue

I'm sure that the moment your baby was born prematurely, your life began to fill with mixed emotions. In the full course of parenting a preemie, you will probably experience every possible feeling that lies between total desperation and absolute elation. I have written this book hoping that, throughout the days ahead, you will be able to use it for intellectual and emotional support as you ride that roller coaster through the highs and lows of preemie care. The information has been presented factually, honestly, openly, and always with a sincere desire to help and comfort you.

As you read, keep in mind that the field of neonatology is rapidly changing and by the time this "up-to-date" text reaches you, there may be newer procedures and treatments available to your child. Always look to your baby's doctors as your first source of information. Use this book as a base of knowledge from which to ask appropriate questions, and also as a constant reminder that parenting a preemie is best done one day at a time.

Appendix A

. . . .

Growth Chart and
Metric Conversion Chart

FAHRENHEIT (F) TO CENTIGRADE (C)

°F	°C	°F	°C	°F	°C	°F	°C
95.0	35.0	98.0	36.7	101.0	38.3	104.0	40.0
95.2	35.1	98.2	36.8	101.2	38.4	104.2	40.1
95.4	35.2	98.4	36.9	101.4	38.6	104.4	40.2
95.6	35.3	98.6	37.0	101.6	38.7	104.6	40.3
95.8	35.4	98.8	37.1	101.8	38.8	104.8	40.4
96.0	35.6	99.0	37.2	102.0	38.9	105.0	40.6
96.2	35.7	99.2	37.3	102.2	39.0	105.2	40.7
96.4	35.8	99.4	37.4	102.4	39.1	105.4	40.8
96.6	35.9	99.6	37.6	102.6	39.2	105.6	40.9
96.8	36.0	99.8	37.7	102.8	39.3	105.8	41.0
97.0	36.1	100.0	37.8	103.0	39.4	106.0	41.1
97.2	36.2	100.2	37.9	103.2	39.6	106.2	41.2
97.4	36.3	100.4	38.0	103.4	39.7	106.4	41.3
97.6	36.4	100.6	38.1	103.6	39.8	106.6	41.4
97.8	36.6	100.8	38.2	103.8	39.9	106.8	41.6

Note: $°C = (°F - 32) \times 5/9$. Centigrade temperature equivalents rounded to one decimal place by adding 0.1 when second decimal place is 5 or greater.

INCHES TO CENTIMETERS

1 inch increments Example: To obtain centimeters equivalent to 22 inches, read "20" on top scale, "2" on side scale; equivalent is 55.9 centimeters.

Inches	0	10	20	30	40
0	0	25.4	50.8	76.2	101.6
1	2.5	27.9	53.3	78.7	104.1
2	5.1	30.5	55.9	81.3	106.7
3	7.6	33.0	58.4	83.8	109.2
4	10.2	35.6	61.0	86.4	111.8
5	12.7	38.1	63.5	88.9	114.3
6	15.2	40.6	66.0	91.4	116.8
7	17.8	43.2	68.6	94.0	119.4
8	20.3	45.7	71.1	96.5	121.9
9	22.9	48.3	73.7	99.1	124.5

One-Quarter (1/4) inch increments Example: To obtain centimeters equivalent to 14¾ inches, read "14" on top scale, "¾" on side scale; equivalent is 37.5 centimeters.

10-15 Inches

	10	11	12	13	14	15
0	25.4	27.9	30.5	33.0	35.6	38.1
1/4	26.0	28.6	31.1	33.7	36.2	38.7
1/2	26.7	29.2	31.8	34.3	36.8	39.4
3/4	27.3	29.8	32.4	34.9	37.5	40.0

16-21 Inches

	16	17	18	19	20	21
0	40.6	43.2	45.7	48.3	50.8	53.3
1/4	41.3	43.8	46.4	48.9	51.4	54.0
1/2	41.9	44.5	47.0	49.5	52.1	54.6
3/4	42.5	45.1	47.6	50.2	52.7	55.2

Note: 1 inch = 2.540 centimeters. Centimeter equivalents rounded one decimal place by adding 0.1 when second decimal place is 5 or greater; for example, 33.48 becomes 33.5.

POUNDS AND OUNCES TO GRAMS

Example: To obtain grams equivalent to 6 pounds, 8 ounces, read "6" on top scale, "8" on side scale; equivalent is 2948 grams.

Ounces	POUNDS 0	1	2	3	4	5	6	7	8	9	10	11	12	13	14
0	0	454	907	1361	1814	2268	2722	3175	3629	4082	4536	4990	5443	5897	6350
1	28	482	936	1389	1843	2296	2750	3203	3657	4111	4564	5018	5471	5925	6379
2	57	510	964	1417	1871	2325	2778	3232	3685	4139	4593	5046	5500	5953	6407
3	85	539	992	1446	1899	2353	2807	3260	3714	4167	4621	5075	5528	5982	6435
4	113	567	1021	1474	1928	2381	2835	3289	3742	4196	4649	5103	5557	6010	6464
5	142	595	1049	1503	1956	2410	2863	3317	3770	4224	4678	5131	5585	6038	6492
6	170	624	1077	1531	1984	2438	2892	3345	3799	4252	4706	5160	5613	6067	6520
7	198	652	1106	1559	2013	2466	2920	3374	3827	4281	4734	5188	5642	6095	6549
8	227	680	1134	1588	2041	2495	2948	3402	3856	4309	4763	5216	5670	6123	6577
9	255	709	1162	1616	2070	2523	2977	3430	3884	4337	4791	5245	5698	6152	6605
10	283	737	1191	1644	2098	2551	3005	3459	3912	4366	4819	5273	5727	6180	6634
11	312	765	1219	1673	2126	2580	3033	3487	3941	4394	4848	5301	5755	6209	6662
12	340	794	1247	1701	2155	2608	3062	3515	3969	4423	4876	5330	5783	6237	6690
13	369	822	1276	1729	2183	2637	3090	3544	3997	4451	4904	5358	5812	6265	6719
14	397	850	1304	1758	2211	2665	3118	3572	4026	4479	4933	5386	5840	6294	6747
15	425	879	1332	1786	2240	2693	3147	3600	4054	4508	4961	5415	5868	6322	6776

Note: 1 pound = 453.59237 grams; 1 ounce = 28.349523 grams; 1000 grams = 1 kilogram. Gram equivalents have been rounded to whole numbers by adding one when the first decimal place is 5 or greater.

Appendix B

. . . .

RESOURCES

Breast-feeding:

For more information about breast-feeding a premature infant, look in the white pages of your phone book for the La Leche League representative nearest you. Ask her for Publication No. 13, *Breastfeeding Your Premature Baby*. Or, write directly to:

> La Leche League International
> P.O. Box 1209
> Franklin Park, IL 60131-8209

The following books may also help you breast-feed your baby successfully:

Brewster, Dorothy Patricia. *You Can Breastfeed Your Baby . . . Even in Special Situations*. Emmaus, Pa.: Rodale Press, 1979.

Eiger, Marvin S., and Olds, Sally Wendkos. *The Complete Book of Breastfeeding*. New York: Workman, 1986.

Grams, Marilyn, M.D. *Breastfeeding Success for Working Mothers*. Sheridan, Wyo.: Achievement Press, 1985.

La Leche League International, Inc. *The Womanly Art of Breastfeeding*. 4th rev. ed. New York: New American Library, 1988.

Messenger, Marie. *The Breastfeeding Book*. New York: Van Nostrand Reinhold Co., 1982.

Diapers:

You can get disposable diapers from:
Premie Pampers
Procter and Gamble Co., Inc.
1-800-543-4932
By the case only (180 diapers)

You can order cloth diapers from:
Preemie Pals
Nancy Nelson
1313 Harrington Ave. S.E.
Renton, WA 98058
1-206-271-0423

Clothing:

Preemie Clothes Patterns:

Claudia Pesek Designs
Precious Preemie Layette
P.O. Box 1184
Grants Pass, OR 97526

Special Patterns by Patricia
1401 34th St.
Anacortes, WA 98221
(For complete set of 4 patterns send $3.95 + .75 postage)

Clothing:

Cot'n tots
22 Lamont Ave.
San Antonio, TX 78209

Sears, Roebuck and Co.
Specialog for Mother and Baby
Catalog Order Department

For a Special Baby
1682 Roxanna St.
New Brighton, MN 55112

Shirey, Inc.
1017 Stanford Ave.
Greenville, TX 75401

I-C Manufacturing Co.
P.O. Box 1060
El Campo, TX 77518

S. Schwab Co., Inc.
P.O. Box 1417
Cumberland, MD 21502

Oh So Small
6432 Pacific Ave.
Tacoma, WA 98408

Tiny Treasures for Molly
and Friends
1060 23rd Ave. S.E.
Minneapolis, MN 55414

Paty, Inc.
4800 W. 34th St.
Houston, TX 77092

Very Important Preemie
312 Broad Ave.
Palisades Park, NJ 07650

Premiers by Alexis
Warren Featherbone Co.
P.O. Box 393
Gainesville, GA 20501

Perinatal Information

For national information on perinatal centers call:
    National Perinatal Information Center
    Providence, RI
    1-401-274-0650

Social Services

Ask your local and state welfare boards for information
about the following departments and programs:

- Bureau of Child Welfare
- Division of Youth and Family Services
- State Department Board of Health

Financial Assistance

Contact your county Board of Social Services. A representative can help you apply for financial aid from the following sources:

- Aid to Families with Dependent Children (AFDC)
- Special Child Health Services (also known as Crippled Children's Program)
  - Women, Infants, and Children (WIC)

Private Organizations

The following organizations may be able to offer you information, social and/or financial assistance. You will find their addresses and phone numbers in the white pages of your phone book.

- Easter Seal Society
- March of Dimes
- United Way

Parent Support Groups

Parent Care, Inc.
101½ S. Union St.
Alexandria, VA 22314-3323

This national organization is made up of professionals and parents who support the establishment and maintenance of parent support groups in intensive care nurseries. They offer educational brochures, a quarterly newsletter, and a referral service that can put you in touch with a parent support group near you.

Neonatal ICU Friends
E. W. Sparrow Hospital
1215 E. Michigan Ave.
Lansing, MI 48912
517-483-2700

This support group comprised of parents and nurses offers information and referral services

Suggested Reading:

The Premature Baby Book
  Helen Harrison
  St. Martin's Press
  New York, 1983

For more information about fetal development:
A Photographic Journey of Discovery Inside the Body
Lennart Nilsson
Little, Brown, and Co.
Boston, 1974

Color Atlas of Life Before Birth: Normal Fetal Development
Marjorie England
Year Book Medical Publishers, Inc.
Chicago, 1983

From Conception to Birth: The Drama of Life's Beginnings
Robert Rugh and Landrum Shettles
Harper & Row
New York, 1971

Glossary

· ·

ABO incompatibility: a blood incompatibility problem that exists when the mother has blood type O, and the baby has blood type A or B. This increases the likelihood of severe newborn anemia and jaundice.

Aid to Families with Dependent Children (AFDC): a government-subsidized program that offers financial assistance to eligible families.

amniocentesis: a procedure for withdrawing amniotic fluid by inserting a needle through the mother's abdomen and into the uterus. Most often this is done to assess lung maturity or to obtain fluid for chromosome composition analysis.

anemia: a medical condition caused by abnormally low concentrations of red blood cells.

antibiotic: a drug that kills bacteria or interferes with its growth.

aorta: the main blood vessel leading from the heart that supplies the body with oxygenated blood.

Apgar score: a means of evaluating, on a scale of 1 to 10, the adaptation of a newborn to the environment outside the uterus immediately after delivery.

apnea: a breathing pause that lasts longer than 15 or 20 seconds.

artery: any blood vessel that leads away from the heart and carries oxygenated blood.

asphyxia: a condition, marked by a serious lack of sufficient oxygen and rising carbon dioxide levels, that affects organ systems and could cause death or major problems if not rapidly treated and reversed.

attending physician: the physician in charge at any given moment.

audiologist: a medical professional who is specially trained to detect, diagnose, and treat individuals with impaired hearing.

Baby Doe case: a 1982 federal legal case that regulates the physician's role in determining the continuance of supportive treatment for most preemies.

bacteria: one-celled organisms that can cause disease.

bagging: pumping air and/or oxygen into the baby's lungs by compressing a bag attached to a mask that covers the baby's nose and mouth.

betamethasone: a steroid drug given to a pregnant woman who is in danger of delivering prematurely. This drug helps the baby's lungs to mature.

bililights: see "phototherapy."

bilirubin: a yellowish red pigment found in small amounts in everyone's blood. Excess amounts sometimes produced in a baby's body cause him to develop jaundice.

blood bank: a store of donated blood to be used in medical procedures.

blood gas analysis: a test to determine the oxygen, carbon dioxide, and acid content of the blood.

blood pressure: the pressure the blood exerts against the walls of the blood vessels. This pressure causes the blood to flow through the arteries and veins.

bonding: a process by which a parent and child become emotionally attached.

bradycardia: a significant drop in the heart rate below the normal rate for that individual. Absolute bradycardia is generally a heartbeat below 90 beats per minute. However, for some babies any significant drop below their normal rate may indicate relative bradycardia, which may be abnormal in certain situations and may have to be treated.

brain bleed: bleeding or hemorrhage into some part of the brain. See "intraventricular hemorrhage."

broviac catheter: a method of giving parenteral nutrition. A narrow flexible tube is inserted into a large vein in the neck or in an arm or leg and threaded through to a large blood vessel near the heart.

BPD: see "bronchopulmonary dysplasia."

bronchial tubes: the tubes that lead from the trachea (windpipe) to the lungs.

bronchopulmonary dysplasia (BPD): a chronic lung disease found in some babies who are on a respirator and/or supplemental oxygen for more than twenty-eight days.

cannula: a method of delivering oxygen. A thin flexible tube is encircled around the baby's face and head and is connected to an oxygen source. A flow meter regulates the amount of oxygen that is given to the baby through the two prongs that extend from the tube into the baby's nostrils.

carbon dioxide (CO_2): a waste product of bodily processes that is carried by the blood to the lungs, where it is exhaled.

cardiology: a branch of medicine dealing with the heart.

cardiopulmonary resuscitation (CPR): a method of reviving a person whose breathing and heartbeat have stopped or slowed abnormally.

catheter: a narrow flexible tube used to administer fluids to the body or to drain fluids from the body.

central nervous system (CNS): the brain and spinal cord.

cerebral palsy (CP): a disorder of the nervous system characterized by problems with muscle movement or tone. Cerebral palsy will not worsen over time.

cervix: the lower part of the uterus that opens into the birth canal.

cesarean birth (C-section): removal of the fetus by means of an incision into the uterus, usually by way of the abdominal wall.

chest physiotherapy (Chest PT): a therapeutic technique in which the care-giver repeatedly taps on the child's back with a small rubber instrument to loosen phlegm, mucus, and other secretions that remain in the lungs.

computerized tomography (CT): a computerized X-ray machine that can take pictures of cross sections of body tissues.

CMV: see "cytomegalovirus."

CNS: see "central nervous system."

colostomy: a surgically created opening in the abdominal wall that allows the colon (the lower section of the large intestine) to empty directly into a waste bag outside the body.

colostrum: the yellowish fluid secreted from the breasts before the mother's milk comes in. It is several times higher in protein than the later milk.

congestive heart failure: the failure of the heart to perform efficiently because of either structural or functional problems.

continuous positive airway pressure (CPAP): a respiratory method that forces a constant flow of air into the lungs through a narrow tube placed in one or both nostrils. Also called positive and expiratory pressure (PEEP).

corrected age: the age a premature baby would be if he had been born on his due date.

CPR: see "cardiopulmonary resuscitation."

cryotherapy: a method of treating retinopathy of prematurity. It is a freezing procedure that stops the abnormal growth of blood vessels that are pulling on the retina.

culture: a method of diagnosis in which samples of body fluids are placed in a specially constructed environment that encourages the growth of infectious organisms, if present, so that they can be analyzed.

cut down: a method of delivering fluids and nourishment by making an incision into the skin, then cutting into a large vein of the arm or leg and threading a narrow tube to a large blood vessel near the heart.

cytomegalovirus (CMV): a type of virus that can be passed on from an infected mother to her unborn child. It can cause severe illness such as hepatitis, encephalitis, or pneumonia and birth defects, such as hydrocephalis or heart abnormalities.

designated donor: a person who donates blood for a specific patient.

developmental pediatrician: a specially trained medical doctor who is primarily concerned with the evaluation of children who are at risk or who may show signs of developmental problems.

developmental problems: these kinds of problems include a lag in motor coordination skills (such as lifting the head up, rolling over, sitting, standing, and walking), hearing or vision impairment, behavioral problems such as extreme irritability or inconsolability, and learning disabilities.

diethylstilbestrol (DES): a synthetic estrogen that was prescribed for women in the 1950s and 1960s to prevent miscarriage. Daughters of these women are now prone to certain types of cancer and to uterine problems, which can include premature delivery.

directed donor: see "designated donor."

diuretic: an agent that increases the production of urine by the kidneys.

early intervention program: a method of physical therapy that may enable a child to utilize his muscles fully and reach his maximal motor potential.

echocardiogram: an ultrasonographic method of recording a picture of the heart as it is produced by the echo of sound waves. This can be used to evaluate both the structure and function of the heart.

electrocardiogram (EKG): a record of the electrical activity of the heart.

electrodes: sensors attached to adhesive pads that are placed on the baby's body to conduct the electrical output of his heartbeat and respiration to a monitor.

electroencephalogram (EEG): a method of recording and analyzing the electrical activity of the brain.

electrolytes: sodium, potassium, chloride, and bicarbonate.

encephalopathy: see "kernicterus."

endotracheal tube: a tube used in the respiratory care of the sickest infants. It is placed into the trachea (windpipe) through the nose or mouth.

evoked potential testing: auditory brain stem response studies, or brain stem auditory evoked response studies, a neurologic diagnostic procedure that determines a baby's potential for hearing.

exchange transfusion: a blood transfusion in which small amounts of the baby's blood are slowly withdrawn and then replaced with equal amounts of donor blood.

extubation: the removal of the endotracheal tube from a patient in order to disconnect him from a respirator.

fellow: a licensed doctor who is completing a two- to three-year training period before taking an exam to become a certified specialist.

fetus: the unborn child in utero from the third month to birth.

fibroids: noncancerous growths in the uterine wall.

flexion: the ability to bend in contrast to extend.

fontanelle: the soft spots lying between the cranial bones of the skull of a newborn.

full-term: an infant born between the thirty-eighth and forty-second week of gestation.

gastrointestinal tract (GI tract): the stomach and intestines.

gavage feeding: see ''naso-gastric.''

gestational age: the age of the fetus and newborn, which is calculated by counting the weeks from the mother's last menstrual period before conception.

GI tract: see ''gastrointestinal tract.''

glucose: a type of simple sugar that supplies the body with energy.

gram: the basic unit of weight in the metric system.

gram-negative organisms: any number of bacteria that may find their way into the baby's respiratory system or blood through a respirator tube during the process of delivery.

Group B Strep infections (GBS): type of bacterial infections that a baby can get from the mother during the birthing process.

heat shield: a device that intensifies the heat from the artificial heat source of the radiant warmer or incubator.

hematocrit: the percentage of red blood cells in the blood.

hemoglobin: the substance in red blood cells that contains iron and carries oxygen.

hemolysis: the rupture of red blood cells.

high-frequency ventilation (HFV): an experimental method of managing a baby's breathing at 500 to 2000 breaths per minute. By drastically increasing the rate of breathing, pressure on the lungs is reduced.

high-risk: a term used to describe persons or situations that require special intervention to prevent a problem from worsening.

hyaline membrane disease: see "respiratory distress syndrome."

hydrocephalus: an abnormal accumulation of spinal fluid in the ventricles of the brain, which is characterized by an abnormal increase in head size and a progressive loss of brain tissue.

hyperalimentation: see "parenteral nutrition."

hyperbilirubinemia: see "jaundice."

hypertension: high blood pressure.

hypotonia: deficient muscle tone.

hypoxia: a lack of sufficient oxygen.

ICN: an abbreviation for "intensive care nursery."

ileostomy: a surgical procedure that creates a diversion of the intestine for the drainage of stool into a bag. This procedure is sometimes used to treat problems such as intestinal obstruction or NEC.

incubator: an enclosed, see-through, temperature-controlled, sometimes double-walled box that gives premature babies environmental protection from bacteria and drafts.

indomethacin: an aspirinlike drug sometimes used to close the patent ductus arteriosus.

Infant Bioethics Committee (Infant Care Review Committees): hospital-based groups comprised of administrators, attending physicians, various medical specialists, and families of patients. When there is a question of continuing or discontinuing aggressive treatment for an infant, this group will meet to evaluate the case and judge the probable outcome. They also formulate guidelines for physicians and families and offer support and educational information.

infection: a condition that occurs when organisms such as bacteria, viruses, and other agents enter the body and change the stability of the vital signs.

infusion pump: a device attached to an intravenous line that carefully regulates in precisely measured amounts the fluids going into a baby's bloodstream.

intensive care nursery (ICN): an area of a Level II or III hospital that is specially equipped with personnel and medical apparatus to provide extensive medical care to sick and premature babies.

intermittent mandatory ventilation (IMV): a respiratory device in which a tube is threaded through the baby's nose or mouth, down the back of the throat, and into the trachea. IMV is most often used in a harmonious pattern with the baby's own breathing rate in order to adequately oxygenate and ventilate the child.

intern: medical doctor who is in his first year of specialty training.

intracranial hemorrhage: see "intraventricular hemorrhage."

intravenous (IV): a tube or needle placed into a surface vein that brings fluids, nourishment, and/or medication into the bloodstream.

intraventricular hemorrhage (intracranial hemorrhage or brain bleed): a medical condition that results from abnormal bleeding on the surface of the brain, in the substance of the brain, or in the brain's central chambers that are continuous with the canal of the spinal cord.

intubation: the insertion of a tube into the trachea (windpipe) through the nose or mouth to allow air to reach the lungs.

in utero: inside the womb.

jaundice (hyperbilirubinemia): a condition that occurs when there is an overabundance of bilirubin in the body.

kernicterus (encephalopathy): an extreme and rare complication of jaundice in which the bilirubin passes into the substance of the brain tissue.

lab technicians: specially trained people who are responsible for running a variety of tests used to monitor and diagnose medical conditions.

lanugo: fine hair that covers the body of a fetus and some preemies.

La Leche League: an international organization dedicated to supporting and encouraging women who want to breast-feed their babies.

large motor skills: skills such as crawling and walking that involve the coordination of large muscle groups.

Lasix: a diuretic drug that may be used to reduce the amount of fluid collecting in the lungs.

lead wires: wires that lead from the electrodes to a monitor.

Level I hospitals: the vast majority of hospitals in America, which have the personnel and facilities to care for routine, uncomplicated labors, deliveries, and full-term healthy newborns.

Level II hospitals: specially designated medical centers that have the personnel and facilities to care for all but the smallest and sickest of premature babies.

Level III hospitals: specially designated medical centers that are often affiliated with a large university. They have a fully equipped intensive care nursery and are staffed with full-time neonatologists and other pediatric specialists.

life-support systems: medical apparatus such as respirators, oxygen delivery systems, IV pumps, etc., that are able to keep people alive when they are incapable of doing so themselves.

lipase: an enzyme found in the body and in breast milk that assists in fat absorption.

LPN: licensed practical nurse.

lumbar puncture: see "spinal tap."

Medicaid: a program of medical assistance for those who are unable to afford regular medical service. It is financed by state and federal governments.

meningitis: inflammation or infection of the spinal cord and the lining of the layers around the brain.

moderately premature: a baby who is born at 35 to 37 weeks gestational age and weighs between 3 pounds 12 ounces and 7 pounds 8 ounces.

monitor: a machine that records information such as heartbeat, body temperature, respiration rate, and blood pressure.

myopia: nearsightedness

naso-gastric tube (NG tube): a narrow, flexible tube that is inserted through the nostril down the esophagus, and into the stomach. It is used to deliver nourishment or to remove air or fluid from the stomach.

necrotizing enterocolitis (NEC): a deterioration of the intestinal tract. It is caused by inflammation of the intestinal tract or decreased blood supply to the bowel. This complication of prematurity generally improves, but it can lead to perforation of the bowel, sepsis, or death.

neonatal period: the first thirty days of life.

neonatologist: a physician who specializes in the development, care, and diseases of newborns.

neurologist: a physician skilled in the diagnosis and treatment of diseases of the nervous system.

noninvasive: without injection, incision, or radiation.

nosocomial infections: bacterial or other types of infections acquired directly from the hospital environment through any point where there is a breakdown in the skin's surface, such as IV or catheter sites, respiratory and feeding tubes, and any surgical incisions. *Staphylococcus epidermidis* and *Staphylo-*

coccus aureus infections are examples of this kind of infection.

obstetrician: a medical doctor who is specially trained to care for a woman's pregnancy, labor, and delivery.

oligohydramnios: too little anmiotic fluid, which can inhibit normal fetal growth.

ophthalmologist: a medical doctor who can diagnose and treat injuries or defects that affect the eyes. He or she can prescribe glasses and medications and can perform surgery.

oro-gastric tube: a narrow, flexible tube that is threaded through the mouth, down the esophagus, and into the stomach. It is used to deliver nourishment or to remove air or fluid from the stomach.

ototoxic antibiotics: drugs used to fight infections. They have the potential to cause hearing problems.

oxygen (O): a gas that is essential to maintaining life. It makes up 21 percent of the room air we breathe.

oxygen hood: a clear plastic box that is placed over the baby's head. It has a tube attached to a unit that supplies varying amounts of oxygen.

oxygen therapy: any method of delivering supplemental oxygen to the infant.

parenteral nutrition (hyperalimentation): a solution fed directly into the baby's bloodstream that gives him necessary nutrients such as carbohydrates, electrolytes, protein, minerals, vitamins, and fat.

parent support groups: organized groups of parents of preemies who offer each other comfort, support, information, and referrals.

patent ductus arteriosus (PDA): a condition in which the blood vessel that connects the aorta (the main artery of the body) and the pulmonary artery (the artery that brings blood to the lungs) does not close as it should shortly after birth.

pediatrician: a physician who specializes in the development, care, and diseases of children.

PEEP: positive end expiratory pressure. See "continuous positive air pressure."

perforated bowel: a hole in the intestine.

perinatal period: the time immediately preceding, during, or after birth.

perinatologist: a medical doctor who specializes in the complications of pregnancy, labor, and delivery.

periodic breathing: breathing interrupted by 10 to 20 second pauses.

peripheral intravenous: a method of supplying nutrition in which a very small needle or plastic catheter is inserted into a surface vein of the arm, leg, or scalp. This method may also be used to supply fluids and medications.

phototherapy (bililights): a mode of treatment for jaundice in which the affected infant is placed under special fluorescent lights that break down the structure of the bilirubin so it can be more easily transported to the liver and then excreted from the body.

physical therapists: medical professionals who will come into the nursery to work with preemies who need extra help with their neuromuscular development. They are also often involved in follow-up developmental care.

placenta: a vascular organ that lines the uterine wall, attaches to the umbilical cord, and delivers nourishment to the fetus.

placental abruption: a condition in which the placenta prematurely pulls away from the wall of the uterus causing painful vaginal bleeding and premature delivery.

placenta previa: a condition in which the placenta covers the cervical opening of the birth canal. It may cause painless vaginal bleeding.

pneumonia: an infection in the area of the lungs involved in the exchange of carbon dioxide and oxygen.

polyhydramnios: excessive amount of anmiotic fluid that puts extra pressure on the uterus and may cause premature birth.

positron emission tomography (PET): a diagnostic technique that can document changes in the metabolism of the brain.

preeclampsia (toxemia): a condition that can cause a reduction in the amount of blood flow through the placenta, which slows down the delivery of vital nutrients to the fetus. It is often associated with high blood pressure, edema, and protein in the urine.

premature infant: a baby born before the thirty-seventh completed week of pregnancy.

premature rupture of the membranes: when the bag of amniotic fluid surrounding the fetus ruptures before the thirty-seventh completed week of gestation.

prenatal: before birth.

primary-care neonatal nurses: medical professionals who have training and experience with the special needs of premature babies.

primary carrier: the health insurance company that takes first responsibility for paying the bills when a family has two health insurance policies.

prognosis: a prediction of the course and end of a disease.

prostaglandins: naturally occurring substances in the body that affect the cardiovascular system by altering the blood flow to a variety of organs. Different classifications of prostaglandins may selectively increase or inhibit the blood flow to a particular organ.

pulmonary artery: the blood vessel that brings blood to the lungs.

pulse oximeter: a device that noninvasively measures the amount of oxygen to the hemoglobin molecules in the blood.

radiant warmer: an open bed with a heat source that allows immediate access to newborn and sick preemies while maintaining a warm air temperature.

radiologist: a medical doctor who has been specially trained to perform and interpret radiographic and ultrasonic procedures.

residents: medical doctors who are in their second or third year of specialty training.

respiration: the act of breathing.

respirator: a machine that provides breathing assistance by supplying and regulating a flow of air, oxygen, and air pressure that goes through a tube threaded through the nose or mouth, down the back of the throat, and into the trachea (windpipe).

respiratory distress syndrome (RDS): a condition (formerly known as hyaline membrane disease) in newborns that causes the child to have difficulty breathing. It is caused by an insufficient supply of a chemical called surfactant that helps expand the small air sacs in the lungs.

respiratory therapists: medical professionals who are trained, certified, and registered to set up, calibrate, monitor, and supervise the use of respiratory equipment.

resuscitation: the act of reviving from apparent death or from unconsciousness.

retina: the lining of the back of the eye that receives visual images.

retinopathy of prematurity (ROP): an eye disease (once called retrolental fibroplasia, or RLF) found primarily in premature infants.

retrolental fibroplasia (RLF): see "retinopathy of prematurity."

Rh factor: a type of identifying protein that may or may not be present in a person's red blood cells.

Rh incompatibility: a blood incompatibility problem in which the mother is Rh-negative, and the baby is Rh-positive. Antibodies from the mother can cause the baby to experience a breakdown of the red blood cells, and very often severe anemia and jaundice.

RhoGAM shots: injections given to a woman with Rh-negative blood. These can be given during her pregnancy or after the birth of her Rh-positive baby.

seizure: abnormal electrical activity of the brain that may be associated with involuntary muscle movements.

sepsis: a medical condition in which there is bacteria in the bloodstream. The bacteria travels in the blood to many parts of the body and causes notable changes in the health condition.

septic shock: a body infection that causes a drop in stability of the vital signs due to a decrease in heart functioning.

shunt: 1. a naturally existing passage between two areas of the body; specifically, the left-to-right or right-to-left shunt through the ductus arteriosus of the heart.

2. a surgically implanted passage between two areas of the body; specifically, the ventriculoperitoneal shunt that drains fluid from the brain ventricles into the abdominal cavity of a child who has hydrocephalus.

sonogram: see "ultrasound."

spinal tap (lumbar puncture): a diagnostic procedure in which a short narrow needle is inserted between two lumbar vertebrae into the area where there is spinal fluid. The spinal fluid is withdrawn for analysis.

stable condition: a medical status at which the baby is breathing without respiratory assistance, is gaining weight, and is self-regulating his body temperature.

Staphylococcus aureus: see "nosocomial infections."

Staphylococcus epidermidis: see "nosocomial infections."

subarachnoid hemorrhage: bleeding in the area around the outside of the brain.

surfactant: a substance formed in the lungs that helps keep the small air sacs expanded and prevents them from collapsing.

surrogate contract: a legal agreement by which a woman agrees to be impregnated and carry a baby for another woman who is unable to carry the baby herself.

swaddling: a method of securely wrapping a baby in a light blanket to soothe and/or restrain him.

term infant: an infant born between the thirty-eighth and forty-second week of gestation.

theophylline: a drug that is sometimes used to treat apnea.

tocolytic drugs: drugs used to stop labor.

toxemia: see "preeclampsia."

trachea: windpipe.

trach tube: a flexible tube that is surgically inserted into the trachea to overcome tracheal obstruction and allow for better respiration.

transfusion: a treatment for anemia in which red blood cells are added directly to the baby's total circulating blood supply through an IV or a catheter.

Trendelenburg bed: a bed that elevates the hips and feet of a woman in premature labor to counter the pull of gravity on the baby.

ultrasound (sonogram): a noninvasive diagnostic technique that records pictures of body tissues and organs through the echoes of high-frequency sound waves.

umbilical catheter (umbilical artery catheter—UAC; umbilical artery line—UAL; umbilical venous catheter—UVC): a narrow, flexible tube inserted through a blood vessel in the baby's navel. When the catheter is placed in an artery, it can be used to draw out blood samples, provide nutrition, infuse blood and medication, and monitor blood pressure. When the catheter is placed in a vein, it is used to give fluids and nutrients and to monitor blood pressure.

vein: a blood vessel leading to the heart.

ventilator: see "respirator."

ventricle: a small chamber; specifically, in the center of the brain or heart.

very premature: a baby born at 30 to 34 weeks gestation and weighing between 2 pounds 3 ounces and 5 pounds 8 ounces.

very-very premature: a baby born at 25 to 29 weeks gestation and weighing between 1 pound 5 ounces and 3 pounds 8½ ounces.

viable: the point at which a fetus is capable of living outside the uterus.

visiting nurses: medical professionals who will come to the home after a preemie's discharge. They are available from four to twenty-four hours a day to help parents manage complicated home-care. These nurses are usually provided as a social service of the local welfare board.

vital signs: respiration, heart rate, body temperature, and blood pressure.

X-ray: a high-energy electromagnetic wave produced by bombarding a target in a vacuum tube with high-velocity electrons. This allows physicians to look at parts of the body that cannot be seen by the naked eye, such as lungs, heart, intestines, and bone.

window period: a space of time during which an infected unit of blood may test free of contamination.

Women, Infants, and Children (WIC): a government-subsidized program that provides food vouchers and financial assistance to eligible families.

Index